Elements of
Medical Genetics

ALAN E. H. EMERY

M.D., Ph.D., D.Sc., F.R.C.P.(E.), M.F.C.M., F.R.S.(E.)
Professor of Human Genetics
University of Edinburgh

FOURTH EDITION

UNIVERSITY OF CALIFORNIA PRESS
BERKELEY AND LOS ANGELES

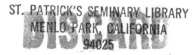

University of California Press
Berkeley and Los Angeles, California

Formerly published as *Heredity, Disease, and Man:
Genetics in Medicine*

ISBN: 0-520-03018-4
Library of Congress Catalog Card Number 68-63004

California Paperback Edition, 1976

Printed in the United States of America

Preface

In preparing this edition, as in previous editions, no attempt has been made to cover all aspects of medical genetics but rather to indicate the ways in which geneticists approach problems in human disease and variation. More emphasis, however, has been placed on the role of genetics in clinical medicine particularly with regard to the prevention of genetic disease.

I am grateful to the publishers of *Lancet,* the *British Medical Journal, Nature* and *Science,* and to Professor Sir Cyril Clarke, Professor J. N. Morris, Dr. A. C. Allison, Dr. S. Abrahamson, Dr. L. L. Heston and Dr. E. R. Huehns for permission to reproduce certain illustrations and published data.

I should also like to thank Professor J. A. Beardmore, Professor J. H. Edwards, Professor H. J. Evans, Professor J. B. Jepson and Dr. Rodney Harris for their comments, criticisms and advice on various sections of the book. Finally I should particularly like to thank Dr. Rosalind Skinner for her help in preparing the manuscript.

1975   ALAN E. H. EMERY

Contents

Chapter		Page
I	The Development of Genetics	1
II	The Chemical Basis of Inheritance	12
III	Biochemical Genetics	27
IV	Chromosomes and Chromosomal Abnormalities	45
V	Developmental Genetics	82
VI	Inheritance in Families	96
VII	Genetic Factors in Some Common Diseases	117
VIII	Pharmacogenetics	139
IX	Population Genetics and Natural Selection	151
X	Radiation and Human Heredity	177
XI	Genetics and the Physician	191
	Glossary	223
	Index	231
	Plates 1 to 13 facing page	136

I

The Development of Genetics

Ideas about heredity can be traced back at least 6000 years by means of stone engravings from Chaldea which depict pedigrees concerning the inheritance of certain characteristics of the mane in horses. With regard to human heredity, the inheritance of the bleeding disorder haemophilia was mentioned in the Talmud some 1500 years ago. However, despite this impressive historical record the nature of conception and explanations of heredity remained largely speculative until comparatively recent times. In fact certain primitive people still consider that sexual intercourse has nothing whatever to do with pregnancy and child bearing.

Aristotle in the third century B.C. suggested that male semen originated from the blood and possessed the ability to give life to the embryo which was formed in the uterus by the coagulation of menstrual blood. This idea was generally accepted for nearly 2000 years until the seventeenth century when William Harvey, who achieved fame for his studies of blood circulation, demonstrated that in deer killed at various times after mating there was never any evidence of coagulation of menstrual blood but that a small embryo developed which gradually increased in size and complexity throughout the whole period of gestation. The credit for first recognizing that the union of egg and sperm is the essential nature of conception is given to a Dutch scientist, Regnier de Graaf. In the latter half of the seventeenth century he described small protuberances on the ovaries of mammals. These protuberances, now called Graafian follicles, contain the unfertilized egg, or ovum. For the first time the idea was put forward that the sperm alone was not the sole hereditary agent thus explaining why the female parent as well as the male parent transmitted characteristics to their offspring. Nevertheless, it was many years before this concept was generally accepted.

Pierre Louis Moreau de Maupertuis was born in France in 1698. Through a fascinating study of him by Professor Bentley Glass we have a picture of a naturalist with views far in advance of his time.

He studied certain hereditary traits in man such as extra fingers (polydactyly) and lack of hair and skin pigmentation (albinism) and from pedigree studies showed that these two conditions were inherited in different ways. He firmly believed that both parents contributed equally to the make-up of their offspring and he provided experimental proof of this from animal breeding experiments. His conception of the structural basis of heredity was novel and in many ways resembled the ideas of Mendel formulated almost 100 years later. Maupertuis proposed that there were hereditary particles; each particle was destined to form a particular body part and each body part was formed by the union of two such particles: one from one parent and one from the other. One particle might dominate the other and so the offspring would come to resemble one parent more than the other.

MENDELISM

The story of our present ideas concerning genetics really starts with the work of the Moravian monk Gregor Mendel, in the latter half of the nineteenth century. Mendel made his far-reaching discoveries through careful and painstaking analysis of the results of crossing varieties of garden pea (*Pisum sativum*). At that time such experiments were not new. T. A. Knight in England in 1823 reported the results of crossing varieties of garden pea. He found that in the first generation, referred to as the *first filial* or F_1 generation, there was dominance of seed colour. That is, if a yellow-seeded plant was crossed with a green-seeded plant all the F_1 plants were yellow seeded, yellowness being dominant to greenness. If these F_1 plants were then self-pollinated (self-fertilized; inbred) the plants in the second generation (F_2) were of both parental colours, that is, green and yellow. Similar results were obtained by others but none of these earlier investigators recorded the actual numbers of the different types of progeny resulting from these various crosses. Prior to Mendel apparently no one thought in terms of inherited units which obeyed statistical laws. This was Mendel's great contribution.

Johann Mendel was born July 22, 1822 in Heinzendorff in Moravia, then part of Austria but now part of Czechoslovakia. He adopted the name Gregor on entering the Augustinian Order in 1843. After becoming a priest he embarked upon the career of school teacher studying physics, mathematics, zoology, and botany at the University of Vienna, but failed to pass the qualifying examination. In 1853 he went to the monastery at Brunn (Brno, now in Czechoslovakia) where his classical experiments on garden peas were carried out. His plant breeding experiments occupied most of his time until he was elected Abbot of the monastery in 1868. Thereafter his time was spent mainly in administrative duties and attempts to persuade the government to exempt monasteries from taxation. He died of Bright's disease (nephritis) on January 6, 1884.

In his plant breeding Mendel selected for study seven pairs of contrasting characters in the garden pea, for example, round or wrinkled seeds, tall or dwarf plants, violet or white flowers, and so on. For each experiment he crossed varieties differing only in one pair of these characters. He classified the hybrids in the F_1 generation and then allowed them to undergo self-pollination and studied the progeny in the F_2 generation. In each of the seven crosses, the plants in the F_1 generation always resembled one of the parental types. For example, when a tall plant was crossed with a dwarf plant all the F_1 offspring were tall. Those characteristics which were manifest in the hybrid were referred to as *dominant* and those which were not manifest in the hybrid were referred to as *recessive*.

The results obtained by allowing self-pollination of the F_1 plants were even more interesting. He found that in the F_2 generation there were individuals manifesting the dominant character but also others manifesting the recessive character. Not only was this true but the dominant and recessive characters in the F_2 generation occurred in a definite ratio of 3 to 1, and no transitional forms were observed. For example, out of 1064 plants in the F_2 generation, 787 were tall and 277 short; a ratio of 2·84 to 1. When the results of his experiments on all the different pairs of contrasting characters were added together the ratio of dominant to recessive was 2·98 to 1. If now the plants exhibiting the recessive character in the F_2 generation were self-pollinated all their progeny in the F_3 generation exhibited the recessive character, that is, short stature. However, if those exhibiting the dominant character in the F_2 generation were self-pollinated, two-thirds yielded offspring which displayed the dominant and recessive characters in the proportion of 3 to 1, and thus resembled the hybrid form in the F_1 generation. When the remaining one-third of the tall plants from the F_2 generation were self-pollinated they yielded offspring which displayed only the dominant character. As Mendel pointed out, the ratio of 3 to 1 in the second generation resolves itself into the ratio of $1 : 2 : 1$ if the apparent dominant forms in this generation are analysed according to the type of offspring they produce when they are self-pollinated. It is possible to explain these results in the following manner. Each individual possesses two ' factors ' which determine a specific characteristic and, as Mendel emphasized, a parent transmits only one of a pair of these factors to any particular offspring. It is purely a matter of chance which of the two factors happens to be transmitted at any one time. This is sometimes referred to as Mendel's 1st law, or the *law of segregation*. In the formation of the sex cells, or gametes, one contrasting character segregates or separates from another. The tall parent plants could be represented as TT, the dwarf parent plants as tt, and the tall hybrid plants in the F_1 generation as Tt. When the latter form gametes, each will contain either the factor T or the factor t. If the hybrid individuals are allowed to undergo self-pollination then union of the two different types of gametes might be expected to occur in the following way:

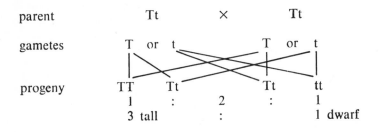

Alternatively the various gametic combinations can be obtained by drawing up what is sometimes referred to as a Punnett's square (after R. C. Punnett, a famous plant geneticist).

		Male gametes	
		T	t
	T	TT	Tt
Female gametes			
	t	Tt	tt

At this point it might be advisable to introduce a few terms. It has already been pointed out that for each physical characteristic or trait, each individual possesses two factors. If these factors are the same then the individual is said to be *homozygous,* but if these factors are different then the individual is said to be *heterozygous* (for example Tt). In the heterozygous state a character which is manifest is dominant; one which is not manifest is recessive. Nearly 50 years ago Johannsen, a Danish botanist, coined the word ' gene ' for these hereditary factors. The genes responsible for contrasting characters are referred to as allelomorphs or alleles for short. Thus in garden pea there are two alleles for stature, one for tallness and one for shortness.

Before Mendel's time it was generally thought that conception involved the mingling of hereditary substances from both parents, each parent transmitting a little of all of its characteristics. But Mendel showed that this was not true. A tall plant did not necessarily transmit some of its tallness to all its progeny. If it were heterozygous then there was an equal chance of it transmitting either the gene for tallness or the gene for shortness. Similarly a person with polydactyly (a dominant factor in man) has an equal chance of transmitting to any particular child either the gene for polydactyly or the gene for normal hands. Each child does not receive from one parent a little bit of each. It is extraordinary that Mendel formulated these ideas without any knowledge of the nature of these hereditary factors or genes.

It has been argued that Mendel's results were almost too good. The numbers of the different types of progeny he obtained were extremely close to the values one would have expected on Mendel's theory. The late Sir Ronald Fisher, an eminent statistician, carefully analysed Mendel's data and concluded that Mendel's experiments were not discoveries but demonstrations of theories which Mendel had in mind when he made the experiments. Be this as it may, the point remains that Mendel's ideas were revolutionary in their day. The validity of his experimental findings has since been confirmed in countless organisms and Mendelism is now the basis of all genetic theory.

Mendel presented the results of his experiments before the Natural History Society of Brunn in 1865 and the following year they were published in the *Transactions* of the Society. However, his work remained largely unknown for nearly 50 years. The reason for this is not at all clear. One suggestion is that the *Transactions of the Natural History Society* of Brunn was an obscure journal, but the journal was at that time not so obscure as might have been expected for it was sent to at least 120 learned societies, academies, and libraries. It seems more likely that scientists in the mid-nineteenth century were simply not prepared for this work. Mendel's contemporaries were preoccupied with Darwin's theory of evolution and the nature of species. Possibly they misinterpreted Mendel's work as a confused attempt to investigate their own problems. Even Carl Nägeli, a world authority on plant hybridization, failed to see the significance of Mendel's results and Nägeli was Mendel's close friend and advisor.

Mendel's laws of heredity remained largely unknown until 1900 when, within the space of a few months, they were independently rediscovered by three biologists: Hugo de Vries, Professor of Botany in the University of Amsterdam, Carl Correns, a botanist at the University of Tübingen, and Erich von Tschermak-Seysenegg, an assistant in the agricultural experimental station at Esslingen near Vienna. All three investigators quite independently arrived at the same conclusions as Mendel had. It is a matter of regret that Mendel died 16 years before his work became generally recognized as being among the most important scientific discoveries of all time.

THE CHROMOSOME THEORY OF INHERITANCE

As interest in ' Mendelian Inheritance ' grew there was much speculation about its physical basis. It was well known that plants and animals were composed of millions of cells, and that each cell contained a nucleus and that within the nucleus were a number of minute threadlike structures called *chromosomes,* so called because of their affinity for certain stains (*chroma*=colour). But until 1903 when Walter S. Sutton and Theodor Boveri independently proposed the chromosome theory of heredity, the association between these minute structures and the phenomenon of inheritance had not been recognized. According to this theory the chromosomes carry the hereditary factors or genes, and the behaviour of the chromosomes at cell division provides the explanation for Mendelian inheritance. The chromosome theory of inheritance is one of the most important concepts in biology, and will be discussed in more detail later. It is interesting to note that Sutton made this major contribution while still a medical student. He later became a surgeon and died at the age of 39 from appendicitis, without ever returning to the field of study which had made him famous.

THE FRUIT FLY

Until 1905, most of the experimental work on genetics had been carried out on plants, but in that year Castle introduced to the laboratory an animal which was to be a major tool in genetic research for many years to come. This was the fruit fly *Drosophila,* which possesses certain distinct advantages for those interested in studying genetics. First, it can be bred in the laboratory with ease. Second, the female produces thousands of eggs during her lifetime and because *Drosophila* develops so rapidly it is possible to study 20 to 25 generations in a year. In man, 25 generations would take about 750 years. Finally, *Drosophila melanogaster,* the species most often studied, has only four pairs of chromosomes, each pair having a distinctive appearance so that it is possible to identify individual chromosomes. In addition, the chromosomes in the salivary glands (and in a few other tissues as well) of *Drosophila* larvae are among the largest known in nature. They are at least 100 times bigger than those in other cells of the body. The reason for their phenomenal enlargement is still not clearly understood. The salivary gland chromosomes possess distinctive patterns of transverse bands which represent the sites of different genes. In some instances it has been possible to localize a particular gene to a very small group of bands or even to a single band.

At Columbia University, Thomas Hunt Morgan and his students Calvin Bridges and A. H. Sturtevant were amongst the first to study the genetics of *Drosophila*. They established the fact that hereditary units or genes were arranged in a particular linear sequence along the length of the chromosomes and cytological studies of the salivary gland chromosomes were often used to confirm the results of their breeding experiments. For his work on *Drosophila,* Morgan was awarded the Nobel Prize in 1934.

THE BEGINNINGS OF HUMAN GENETICS

We might now turn to the work of some of the founders of human genetics. To be sure, interest in human genetics did not spring up overnight. We have seen how Maupertuis studied the inheritance of albinism and polydactyly in the eighteenth centry. Otto's account in 1803 of haemophilia in a New Hampshire family was apparently the earliest clear description of the clinical features and mode of inheritance of this disease: it was transmitted by healthy carrier females to their sons but never by an affected father to his son. A trait which is inherited in such a manner we call sex-linked. This will be discussed later.

Until the beginning of the present century most investigators of human heredity were mainly interested in tracing pedigrees. Other aspects of human genetics received very little attention, except for a few studies on the effects of cousin marriages (= consanguineous marriages). One of the first scientists to become interested in the effects of inbreeding was Charles Darwin, who himself married a first cousin. The results of his plant breeding experiments led him to conclude that the progeny of crosses between unrelated organisms (outbreeding) were more vigorous than the progeny of crosses between related organisms (inbreeding). The French neurologist Ménière in 1856 suggested that in man deaf mutism was more common in the children of cousin marriages. All in all our knowledge of inheritance in man had progressed very little by the end of the nineteenth century.

Johannsen was the first to make clear the distinction between *genotype,* meaning the genetic constitution, and *phenotype,* meaning the appearance of an individual which results from the interaction of environment on the genotype. Thus a garden pea plant may have the genotype Tt but have a dwarfed phenotype because it grew in a shaded or poorly irrigated location. In man, the distinction between the effects of nature and nurture were made clear for the first time in 1875 by Sir Francis Galton who, like his eminent cousin Charles Darwin, began his career as a medical student but later on forsook medicine after being left a substantial legacy. Galton argued that since identical twins have the same genetic constitution, any difference between them must be due to environment, that is, identical twins have the same genotype but may have different phenotypes because of having grown up in different environments. Galton was especially interested in the inheritance of physique and special talents. In pursuing this interest, he studied families of wrestlers in the North of England. He realized, however, the unsatisfactory nature of qualitative estimates of such talents and the importance of quantifying the characteristics under study. As a means of estimating the degree of resemblance between various relatives he introduced to genetics the statistical concept of the regression coefficient. Galton's work formed a cornerstone for many future investigators interested in the more mathematical aspects of human heredity.

Galton had many interests and among them was the advancement of the idea of hereditary improvement of men and animals by such methods as selective breeding for which he coined the word *eugenics.* Over the years a eugenics movement developed which had fervent followers both in Europe and the United States. It seemed reasonable at the time that a desirable aim of human geneticists should be the improvement of the human species by selective breeding. For many years, therefore, human genetics and eugenics were linked in people's minds, but even today our knowledge of human genetics is too rudimentary to advocate drastic eugenic policies. What information we do have suggests that such measures would be largely inadequate anyway. This is not to say, however, that there is no place for warning those who carry harmful hereditary factors of the risks of having affected children, and of explaining the importance of family limitation in such cases.

GENETICS AND DISEASE

One of the greatest proponents of Mendelism was William Bateson. The story is told that while he was on a train to London to present a paper before the Royal Horticultural Society on the results of his own plant breeding experiments, he read Mendel's paper for the first time and from then on became a fervent disciple of Mendelism. He translated the paper from German into English and had it published in the *Journal of the Royal Horticultural Society* of 1900. Immediately following the rediscovery of Mendelism in 1900 much effort was spent in attempts to apply these findings to man. Unfortunately many of the earlier investigators over-simplified things in order to make their observations agree with Mendel's concepts of dominance and recessiveness. For example, Davenport, who founded the Eugenics Record Office in the United States and was a prominent figure among human geneticists during the first quarter of the twentieth century, firmly believed that mental deficiency in general was inherited as a recessive trait. This is not true. There are many forms of mental deficiency, and although a few are inherited as Mendelian traits, most cases are due to the effects of many genes, so-called multifactorial inheritance. These early investigators not only believed that many human diseases were explicable in terms of the effects of single genes but that all disorders were either due to heredity or environment. This again was an oversimplification.

Nowadays we believe that both hereditary and environmental factors play a part in the causation of the vast majority of diseases, though in some cases one may appear to be more important than the other.

Alkaptonuria is a very rare condition in which affected persons excrete dark-coloured urine. The disease is usually recognized in infancy because the napkins are dark stained and in fact washing with soap tends to make these stains even more intense. The dark colour is due to the presence of homogentisic acid which in normal people is broken down and so does not appear in the urine. The disease is not serious and apart from arthritis, which may ensue as a complication later in life, the disorder is harmless and not incapacitating. In 1901, in a paper read before the Royal Medical and Chirurgical Society in London, Sir Archibald Garrod described four families in which 11 persons had alkaptonuria and no less than three affected individuals were the offspring of first cousin marriages. In each case the parents of affected individuals were apparently normal. Bateson suggested to Garrod that alkaptonuria was probably a rare recessive disorder because, he argued, since first cousins are more likely to share the same genes inherited from a common grandparent, so a high frequency of consanguineous marriages would be expected among the parents of individuals homozygous for a rare gene. This is exactly what Garrod had found in the families with alkaptonuria. In general terms, the rarer a recessive disorder the more often it will be found that the parents of affected individuals are cousins.

Until Garrod's discoveries, genetics had been largely concerned with the inheritance of structural or other obvious abnormalities such as polydactyly in man or flower colour in peas. The novel and important point made by Garrod was that in alkaptonuria there was an inherited disorder involving a chemical process or, as Garrod preferred to call it, an *inborn error of metabolism*. This was the beginning of biochemical genetics and the idea that genes control the synthesis of enzymes, which in turn are responsible for carrying out specific biochemical processes. Beadle and Tatum provided experimental evidence for these ideas from breeding experiments with the bread mould *Neurospora crassa*. Their work was of such importance that they were awarded the Nobel Prize in Medicine and Physiology in 1958.

At about the same time that Garrod was making his important observations on the inheritance of alkaptonuria and certain other biochemical abnormalities in man, Karl Landsteiner discovered the ABO blood groups. This discovery was the prelude to an important branch of human genetics, namely blood-group genetics.

Finally in 1956, Tjio and Levan, and independently Ford and Hamerton, clearly demonstrated for the first time that the number of chromosomes in man was 46 and not 48 as was previously believed. The great contribution made by these investigators was the introduction of improved methods for studying chromosomes. Until then it had been very difficult to study human chromosomes because of their small size. With the new techniques it was possible to separate them and observe them more accurately. This was largely the reason for the ' chromosome breakthrough ' in 1959 when Lejeune in Paris and Ford and Jacobs in Britain demonstrated that in patients with Down's syndrome (mongolism) and in those with various abnormalities of sexual development there were clearly recognizable, specific, chromosome aberrations.

This historical introduction of necessity has been brief and rather sketchy, but nevertheless certain basic ideas should now be evident. First, the general principles of heredity as discovered by Mendel in garden peas, are applicable to all living creatures, including man. Second, unlike animal genetics, the study of human genetics is inherently difficult because we cannot carry out breeding experiments. On the other hand we know more about the biochemistry and physiology of man than we do about any other organism. Third, some of the most profound observations in human genetics have been made on rare and obscure diseases.

FURTHER READING

Boyer, S. H. (ed.) (1963). *Papers on Human Genetics.* Englewood Cliffs, N.J.: Prentice-Hall.
Carlson, E. A. (1966). *The Gene: a Critical History.* Philadelphia: Saunders.
Dunn, L. C. (1962). Cross currents in the history of human genetics. *Am. J. hum. Genet.* **14**, 1–13.
Dunn, L. C. (1965). *A Short History of Genetics.* New York: McGraw-Hill.
Fisher, R. A. (1936). Has Mendel's work been rediscovered? *Ann. Sci.* **1**, 115–137.
Garrod, A. E. (1902). The incidence of alkaptonuria: a study in chemical individuality. *Lancet* **ii**, 1616-1620.
Gasking, E. B. (1959). Why was Mendel's work ignored? *J. Hist. Ideas.* **20**, 60–84.
Glass, B. (1947). Maupertuis and the beginnings of genetics. *Q. Rev. Biol.* **22**, 196–210.
McKusick, V. A. (1960). Walter S. Sutton and the physical basis of Mendelism. *Bull. Hist. Med.* **34**, 487–497.
Needham, J. (1959). *A History of Embryology.* 2nd ed. Cambridge University Press.
Peters, J. A. (1959). *Classic Papers in Genetics.* Englewood Cliffs, N.J.: Prentice-Hall.
Platt, R. (1959). Darwin, Mendel and Galton. *Med. Hist.* **3**, 87–99.
Sorsby A. (1965). Gregor Mendel. *Br. Med. J.* **1**, 333–338.
Stern, C. and E. R. Sherwood (1966). *The Origin of Genetics.* San Francisco: Freeman.
Sturtevant, A. H. (1965). *A History of Genetics.* New York: Harper & Row.

II

The Chemical Basis of Inheritance

How does a gene determine a particular characteristic? For example, how does one gene determine eye colour and yet another determine whether a person will have extra fingers? What is the chain of events which leads from the gene to the final product? These are difficult questions to answer and are the main concern nowadays of much biological research. The purpose of this chapter is to answer some of these questions but it should be realized that our understanding of gene action is still very far from being complete.

THE NUCLEUS

Within each cell of the body are located the cytoplasm and a dark-staining body, the nucleus (fig. 1). The cytoplasm used to be considered merely a fluid which bathed the nucleus but this is now believed to be an oversimplification. The cytoplasm certainly is semifluid in consistency but it has within itself a complex arrangement of very fine tubes which open onto the surface of the cell (= *endoplasmic reticulum*). These tubes are probably involved in conducting nutrients from the outside to the inside of the cell and are

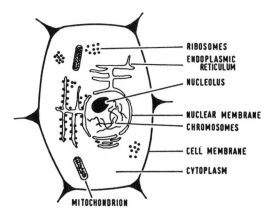

RIBOSOMES
ENDOPLASMIC RETICULUM
NUCLEOLUS
NUCLEAR MEMBRANE
CHROMOSOMES
CELL MEMBRANE
CYTOPLASM
MITOCHONDRION

Figure 1. A schematic diagram of an animal cell.

particularly well developed in the cells of the pancreas. Also situated within the cytoplasm are small bodies concerned with cell respiration (*mitochondria*) and others, even more minute, concerned with protein synthesis (*ribosomes*). Both these structures are extremely small and their study has only been possible recently with the advent of the electron microscope. The nucleus itself is surrounded by a membrane which separates it from the cytoplasm and within the nucleus are the chromosomes which bear the genes.

DNA AND THE CHEMISTRY OF GENES

In 1869 a young German chemist named Friedrich Miescher carried out experiments on the chemical composition of cell nuclei. He obtained pus from used surgical dressings and subjected it to chemical analysis. Pus is known to be rich in nuclei and this was the reason for using it for his work. After much painstaking effort Miescher's analysis revealed a substance which was neither carbohydrate, protein, nor fat. At that time it was considered unique among organic compounds because it contained a very high proportion of phosphorus. Since it was obtained from nuclei he called it *nuclein* but it was later renamed nucleic acid when its acidic properties were recognized. Despite the fact that these experiments had shown that nucleic acid was clearly the chemical substance in nuclei, most biochemists continued to believe for many years that protein was *the* basic substance of life. The results of certain experiments were to show that this view was incorrect.

Two forms of pneumonia-causing bacteria (pneumococci) can be recognized by the appearance of their colonies when grown in the laboratory. These two forms are referred to as rough (R) and smooth (S). Both forms normally breed true, but in 1928 it was shown by Griffith that if a colony of the S form were killed by boiling and the remains were mixed with living R bacteria, some of the latter were transformed into S bacteria. These latter bred true as did the remaining R bacteria.

Dead S + Living R → Living S + Living R

This means that a substance in the dead S bacteria had been transferred to and changed the genetic nature of some of the R bacteria. This significant experiment drew little attention at the time but in 1944 these experiments were repeated by Avery, MacLeod, and McCarty at the Rockefeller Institute. Their investigations showed that the substance which brought about the change in the pneumococci was nucleic acid. They purified extracts from the dead S bacteria and showed the transformation of R to S could be brought about by using a solution of the nucleic acid only.

A second experiment which proved that nucleic acid was the essential component of hereditary material was made by Hershey and Chase in 1952. They worked on minute virus particles which attacked bacteria cells. These bacterial viruses are called bacteriophages, or phages for short (fig. 2). Each phage particle consists of a

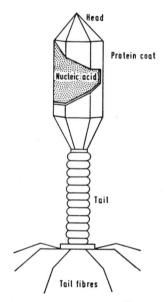

Figure 2. A bacteriophage.

head and a tail and has a protein coat which surrounds a central core of nucleic acid. By means of its tail it becomes attached to a bacterium and after infection many new phage particles, complete with protein coats, are formed within the bacterial cell. Eventually the new particles burst out of the host cell and invade other bacteria. By an ingenious technique Hershey and Chase labelled the protein coat of phage particles with radioactive sulphur, and the nucleic acid within the phage particles with radioactive phosphorous. There is no sulphur in nucleic acid and almost no phosphorus in protein. They then allowed these labelled bacteriophages to infect bacteria. Later they separated the bacteria from the remains of the bacteriophages by means of a Waring Blendor. When the infected bacteria were analysed Hershey and Chase found that only the radioactive phosphorus of the nucleic acid had entered the bacterial cells, and not the radioactive sulphur. Since bacteriophage particles, *complete with their protein coats*, are formed within infected bacterial cells, and since only nucleic acid enters the bacterial cell, this means that genetic information necessary for the synthesis of protein is carried only by nucleic acid. This and the previous evidence clearly showed that genetic information is carried by nucleic acid.

Let us now examine the structure of nucleic acid for help in understanding how genetic information is stored. Nucleic acid is a complex substance and its composition and structure have taken many years to determine. It is composed of long chains of molecules called nucleotides. Each nucleotide is composed of a nitrogenous base, a sugar molecule, and a phosphate molecule. The nitrogenous bases are called purines and pyrimidines. The purines include adenine and guanine; the pyrimidines include cytosine, thymine and uracil. There are two different nucleic acids. One contains the sugar ribose and is therefore called *ribonucleic acid* or RNA. The other contains a slightly different sugar called deoxyribose and is therefore called *deoxyribonucleic acid* or DNA. RNA is found mainly in the nucleolus (a structure within the nucleus) and the cytoplasm, there being very little in the chromosomes. DNA on the other hand is found mainly in the chromosomes. Both nucleic acids contain cytosine and have the same purine bases, but whereas thymine occurs only in DNA, uracil occurs only in RNA.

Now if genes are composed of DNA it is necessary that the latter should have a structure sufficiently versatile to account for the great variety of different genes and yet at the same time be able to reproduce itself in such a manner that an identical replica of itself is formed at each cell division. In 1953, studies of DNA by M. H. F. Wilkins, F. H. C. Crick, and J. D. Watson based on X-ray diffraction proposed a structure for the DNA molecule which fulfilled all the essential requirements. For their work Wilkins, Watson, and Crick were awarded the Nobel Prize for Medicine and Physiology.

Watson and Crick suggested that the DNA molecule is composed of two chains of nucleotides arranged in a double helix. The backbone of each chain is formed by sugar-phosphate molecules and the two chains are held together by hydrogen bonds between the nitrogenous bases which point in toward the centre of the helix. The arrangement of the bases is not random: a purine in one chain always pairs with a pyrimidine in the other chain. There is also specific base pairing: guanine in one chain always pairs with cytosine in the other chain and adenine always pairs with thymine (fig. 3). This model of the DNA molecule is referred to as the Watson-Crick model and a considerable body of experimental evidence in its

favour has accumulated over the last 20 years. Much of this evidence
has come from work on bacteria and bacteriophage.

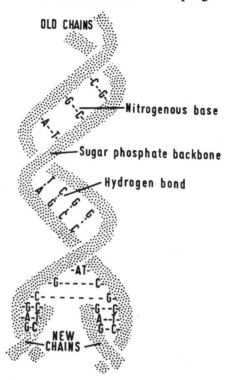

Figure 3. The DNA molecule, composed of two chains of nucleotides, the
backbone of each chain being formed by sugar-phosphate molecules. During
replication the two chains separate while complementary chains are being
synthesized.

The Watson-Crick model provides an answer to the vexing question of how genetic information is transmitted from one cell generation to another. It is postulated that at nuclear division the two
strands of the DNA molecule separate and as a result of specific
base pairing, each chain then builds its complement. In this way
when cells divide, genetic information would be conserved and transmitted unchanged to each daughter cell. There is good evidence
that the DNA molecule does in fact replicate in this manner.

The idea that each chromosome is composed of a single Watson-
Crick double helix of DNA is attractive, but is perhaps an oversimplification. The width of a chromosome is very much greater

than the diameter of a DNA helix. Also if each chromosome represents only one double helix of DNA, the helices would have to be
extremely tightly coiled because the amount of DNA in each nucleus
is such that in man the total length of his chromosomes when extended would amount to several yards! In fact the *total* length of the
human chromosome complement is less than half a millimetre. If the
DNA molecule is so highly coiled then it is necessary to explain
how this phenomenal amount of coiling is undone each time a
chromosome replicates. The mechanical problems involved in un-
winding such a coil would be enormous. The DNA molecule almost
certainly has a structure as represented in the Watson-Crick model.
The difficulty lies in relating this to the known structure and behaviour of the intact chromosome. A considerable gap in our knowledge exists between what is known at the molecular level and what
is visualized at the microscopic level. There is obviously something
fundamental about the structure of chromosomes which we still do
not understand.

THE GENETIC CODE

To account for the great variety of different genes on the basis of the
Watson-Crick model of DNA is not so difficult as it may appear at
first. There are 20 *different* amino acids in protein. Since the primary
action of the gene is to synthesize protein, it can be imagined that
all the varieties of different genes might be reduced to 20 different
arrangements within the DNA molecule. This forms the basis of the
so-called genetic code.

Genetic information is stored within the DNA molecule in the
form of a triplet code, that is, a sequence of three bases determines
the structure of one amino acid. The reason for believing this is as
follows. Since only 20 *different* amino acids are found in proteins
and since the DNA molecule contains four nitrogenous bases,
obviously each base cannot specify one amino acid, for this would
account for only four amino acids. If two bases specified one amino
acid there would be 4^2 or 16 possible combinations. This is also
not enough. However if three bases specified one amino acid then
the possible number of combinations of four bases taken three at a
time would be 4^3 or 64. This is more than enough to account for
all the 20 known amino acids. The triplet of nucleotide bases which
codes for one amino acid is sometimes called a *codon*.

The information stored in the code is in some way transmitted
from the DNA of the gene to a particular type of RNA, so-called
messenger-RNA. For some time it has been known that cells which

synthesize large amounts of protein, such as liver cells, are rich in RNA. The relationship between RNA and protein synthesis is clearly shown in experiments with certain viruses such as the

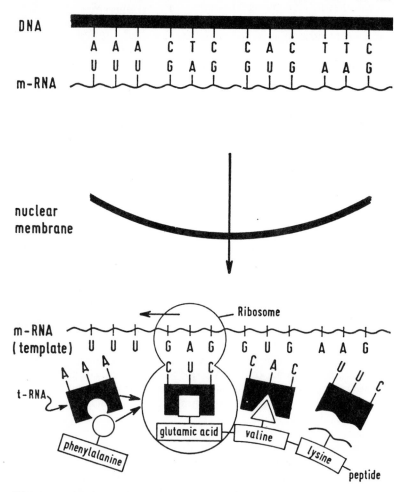

Figure 4. Diagrammatic representation of the way in which genetic information is translated into protein synthesis.

tobacco mosaic virus. Plant foliage infected with this virus develops a characteristic mottled appearance. The virus contains a central mass of RNA surrounded by a protein coat. When the RNA is separated from the protein coat it is found that the coat alone is not infective. However, if the RNA alone is applied to the leaves of a healthy plant, it soon develops the disease and whole virus particles, complete with their particular protein coats, can be recovered from the diseased plant. The process whereby information is transmitted from DNA to messenger-RNA is called ' *transcription* ' and is not yet clearly understood. But the way in which genetic information from messenger-RNA is ' *translated* ' into protein synthesis is better understood (fig. 4).

Each messenger-RNA is formed by a particular gene, such that every base in the messenger-RNA molecule is complementary to a corresponding base in the DNA of the gene: cytosine with guanine, thymine with adenine but adenine with *uracil* since the latter replaces thymine in RNA. The messenger-RNA then migrates out of the nucleus into the cytoplasm where it becomes associated with the ribosomes which are the site of protein synthesis. A group of ribosomes associated with the same molecule of messenger-RNA are referred to as polyribosomes or polysomes. In the ribosomes the messenger-RNA forms the template or mould for sequencing particular amino acids and is therefore sometimes referred to as template-RNA. In the cytoplasm is yet another form of RNA called transfer—or soluble—RNA. For the incorporation of amino acids into a polypeptide chain, the amino acids must first be activated by reacting with ATP. Each activated amino acid then attaches itself to one end of a particular transfer-RNA. The other end of the transfer-RNA molecule consists of three bases which combine with complementary bases on the messenger-RNA. Thus a particular triplet on the messenger-RNA is related through transfer-RNA to a specific amino acid. The ribosome moves along the messenger-RNA in a zipper-like fashion, the amino acids linking up to form a polypeptide chain (fig. 4). When the completed polypeptide chain is released, the ribosome reattaches itself to a new starting point on a messenger-RNA molecule.

CRACKING THE CODE

The first successful attempt to find the key to the genetic code and so discover which triplet stands for which amino acid was made by Nirenberg and Matthaei in 1961. These two investigators, working at the National Institutes of Health in the United States, found that under certain conditions when they added RNA containing only the nitrogenous base uracil (U) to a mixture of amino acids, enzymes, and ribosomes, a simple protein was synthesized. Thus they had been able to imitate in the test tube the process which takes place in the intact cell. What is more, the protein they synthesized contained only the amino acid phenylalanine, though all the other amino acids were present and available in the mixture. In other words the triplet UUU is equivalent to the amino acid phenylalanine. The next step was to introduce into the RNA molecule containing uracil (U), an occasional adenine (A) so that the nucleic acid consisted mainly of U but with an occasional A occurring at random: UUUAUUUUAUUAUUU. . . . In such a chain most of the triplets would be UUU but a few might be UUA, UAU, or AUU depending on where the chain was broken. Using such a nucleic acid it was found, as might be expected, that the resultant protein was composed mainly of phenylalanine but a few other amino acids had also been incorporated corresponding to the additional triplets containing adenine. These other amino acids were leucine, isoleucine, and tyrosine. By similar experiments with various refinements, triplet codes have been assigned to all 20 amino acids. Some amino acids are coded by more than one triplet and so the code is sometimes said to be *degenerate* (table I).

There remains another problem worth considering, namely, whether the triplet code is overlapping or not. If the sequence of bases in a particular template-RNA is UAAGCAUAGG, then the different possible triplets are UAA, AAG, AGC, GCA, CAU, AUA, UAG, AGG. Obviously if the triplets overlap, chaos would result if different transfer-RNA's could attach themselves anywhere. Dintzis has shown experimentally that this does not happen. Transfer-RNA's, with their amino acids, become attached in sequence along the messenger-RNA starting at one end and gradually extending to the other. In the example given above one transfer-RNA would become attached to UAA and when this was done another would become attached to GCA and so on along the length of the messenger-RNA. What happens if, as in the case of a mutant gene, the order of bases at a particular point in the RNA molecule is changed? There are two possibilities. Either the resulting code is read as ' non-sense ' and no amino acid is produced or the resulting code is read as ' mis-sense ' in which case a different amino acid is substituted in the protein molecule with the result that the abnormal protein may have altered or even no biological activity. For example, it may have lost its enzymatic properties. *Ochre* and *Amber* (table I) are two codons found in micro-organisms which do not code for any amino acid (non-sense mutations) and are believed to signal the termination of a peptide chain. Most of the abnormal haemoglobins (p. 36) are the result of mis-sense mutations as are probably many of the inborn errors of metabolism·

Table I. Genetic code in terms of RNA triplets (or codons)

1st base	2nd base				3rd base
	U	C	A	G	
U	Phenylalanine	Serine	Tyrosine	Cysteine	U
	Phenylalanine	Serine	Tyrosine	Cysteine	C
	Leucine	Serine	*Ochre	* —	A
	Leucine	Serine	*Amber	Trytophan	G
C	Leucine	Proline	Histidine	Arginine	U
	Leucine	Proline	Histidine	Arginine	C
	Leucine	Proline	Glutamine	Arginine	A
	Leucine	Proline	Glutamine	Arginine	G
A	Isoleucine	Threonine	Asparagine	Serine	U
	Isoleucine	Threonine	Asparagine	Serine	C
	Isoleucine	Threonine	Lysine	Arginine	A
	Methionine	Threonine	Lysine	Arginine	G
G	Valine	Alanine	Aspartic acid	Glycine	U
	Valine	Alanine	Aspartic acid	Glycine	C
	Valine	Alanine	Glutamic acid	Glycine	A
	Valine	Alanine	Glutamic acid	Glycine	G

* Chain termination.

In 1970, Khorana and his colleagues succeeded in synthesizing a gene *de novo*. They assembled the 77 base pairs of the gene which codes for the production alanine transfer RNA in yeast. But this artificial gene, while structurally correct, was non-functional both in cells and in the test tube mainly because it did not contain the initiator and terminator signals that start and regulate the synthesis of transfer RNA. However, three years later Nobel laureate Khorana succeeded in synthesizing the first wholly artificial gene with the potential for functioning inside a living cell. This was the 126-unit DNA fragment which codes for the production of tyrosine transfer RNA in *Escherichia coli*. Granted that this is not a gene which codes for protein, the discovery is a major advance which may lead to the eventual synthesis of a gene related to an inherited metabolic disorder in man.

RNA-DIRECTED DNA SYNTHESIS

Until recently is was generally believed that genetic information was transferred from DNA to RNA and thence translated into protein synthesis. However, there is increasing evidence, which has come mainly from the study of viruses, that genetic information may occasionally flow in the reverse direction (i.e. from RNA to DNA). This is referred to as RNA-directed DNA synthesis. It has been suggested by Temin, who has been largely responsible for this work, that regions of DNA in normal cells serve as templates for the synthesis of RNA which in turn then acts as a template for the synthesis of DNA which later becomes integrated with the cellular DNA. He suggests that the resultant amplification of certain regions of DNA may be an important factor in embryonic differentiation and possibly in the pathogenesis of cancer.

CONTROL OF PROTEIN SYNTHESIS

Structural genes

Genes are responsible for the synthesis of protein, and a change (mutation) of a base pair of the DNA molecule may have diverse effects on the corresponding protein. Firstly the change may result in another triplet which codes for the same amino acid. In this case there will be no alteration to the properties of the resulting protein. Perhaps 20 to 25 per cent of all possible single base changes are of this type. Secondly, in about 70 to 75 per cent of cases, a single base mutation results in a change in the triplet code producing a different amino acid and the synthesis of an altered protein. This may so affect the molecular structure of the protein that there is a gross reduction or even a complete loss of biological activity. Alternatively the result may not be so much a quantitative as a qualitative change in the protein such that it retains its normal biological activity (e.g. enzyme activity) but differs in such characteristics as its mobility on electrophoresis, its pH optimum, or its stability so that it is more rapidly broken down *in vivo*. Thirdly, in about 2 to 4 per cent of single base changes, the result is a triplet which codes for the termination of a peptide chain. In most cases the shortened chain is unlikely to retain normal biological activity particularly if the termination occurs, for example, before the active centre of an enzyme molecule. Finally, a gene mutation may involve more than a single base in the DNA sequence. It may involve such rearrangements as loss or duplication of part of the sequence with corresponding changes in biological activity. Thus in the inborn errors of metabolism, the level of a particular enzyme may be reduced because it is not synthesized, or it is synthesized but has reduced activity or increased instability. Rarely a gene mutation may lead to the *increased* synthesis of an enzyme resulting in *increased* activity (e.g. the Hektoen variant of G-6-P.D.). There is also evidence that in some genetic disorders though a specific protein may be synthesized, and its presence can be demonstrated by immunological methods, the protein is functionally inactive. This seems to be so in most patients with haemophilia (p. 29).

Control genes

So far we have been discussing what are referred to as *structural* genes, that is genes responsible for the synthesis of specific proteins and enzymes. We shall now consider the action of *control* genes.

One gene may modify the effects of another gene. This is illustrated in the rare case in which persons appear to have blood-group O, yet family studies reveal that they must carry the gene for group A (or B). The first family in which this was described was in Bombay and so it is called the Bombay phenomenon. It is believed to be due to the effects of a rare gene which in the homozygous state suppresses the AB blood-group genes. Other examples of modifier genes are known but whether there is interaction of gene products rather than interaction between the genes themselves is not clear. Direct interaction between genes is believed to occur in the case of so-called control genes.

In 1961, as a result of their extensive work on the genetics of the bacterium *Escherichia coli,* Jacob and Monod of the Pasteur

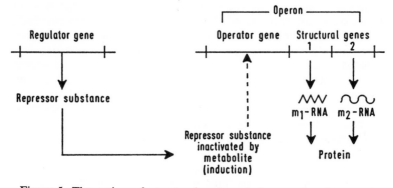

Figure 5. The action of structural and control genes (regulator and operator genes).

Institute postulated that besides structural genes there are *control* genes (regulator and operator genes) which are not directly concerned with the synthesis of specific proteins but regulate the activity of structural genes and therefore control the *amount* of gene product.

According to Jacob and Monod a unit of gene action is the *operon* which consists of an operator gene and the adjacent structural genes whose action the operator gene controls. The operator gene in its turn is controlled by a regulator gene which is not necessarily

Table II. *Various types of regulator and operator gene mutations and their expression in the homozygote or heterozygote*

Mutation	Type	Effect	Function	Expression
Regulator	regulator negative	non-functioning regulator gene	↑	homozygote
	super-repressor	altered repressor not inactivated by inducer	↓	heterozygote
Operator	operator negative	non-functioning operator gene	↓	homozygote
	constitutive operator	operator gene insensitive to repressor	↑	heterozygote

close to the operator gene. The regulator gene synthesizes a substance (' repressor ') which inhibits the operator gene (fig. 5). Thus when the regulator gene is functioning proteins are not synthesized by the associated structural genes. The latter only function when the regulator is ' switched off ' by the repressor being inactivated by a specific metabolite referred to as an *inducer*. In man possible examples of operons are those inherited disorders in which there is a deficiency of more than one enzyme. For example, sucrose intolerance, a recessive disorder characterized by severe attacks of diarrhoea, is associated with deficiencies of intestinal sucrase, maltase and isomaltase, and oroticaciduria, a recessive disorder with severe megaloblastic anaemia in which two successive enzymes in pyrimidine biosynthesis are deficient.

Various types of mutations of regulator or operator genes have been identified in haploid (having only one set of chromosomes) micro-organisms, and the possible effects in diploid organisms are summarized in table II. For example, in a regulator negative type of mutation, the regulator gene is non-functioning, the operator gene is therefore no longer repressed and protein synthesis is increased. In a diploid organism this type of mutation would be expressed only in the homozygote since the repressor substance made by the regulator allele on the homologous chromosome is sufficient to repress protein synthesis on both chromosomes. Alternatively a mutation which results in the synthesis of an altered repressor, such that it is no longer inactivated by an inducer, will lead to a decrease in protein synthesis and since the repressor is diffusible, it will exert its effect on the homologous chromosome and will therefore be manifest in the heterozygote. These various types of mutations have been discussed in detail by Dreyfus (1969). However, there is so far little evidence for the existence of control gene mutations in man and most hereditary biochemical abnormalities, usually inherited as autosomal recessive traits, are believed to be due to mutations of structural genes. The subject has been dealt with in some detail only to emphasize that mechanisms other than structural gene mutations and chromosome abnormalities may account for certain genetic disorders. It has been suggested, for example, that a regulator negative type of mutation may account for congenital erythropoietic porphyria (a recessive disorder characterized by excess production of porphyrins with purple urine, haemolytic anaemia and skin photosensitivity) and a super-repressor type mutation for von Willebrand's disease (a dominant disorder with a deficiency of anti-haemophilic globulin and a vascular abnormality leading to a prolonged bleeding time).

The Jacob and Monod model of gene control mechanisms is now widely accepted. However, the theory does not explain the coordinated activity of non-adjacent operons. The so-called Britten-

Davidson model is a new theory which attempts to explain how widely separated genes might be controlled by diffusing ' activator ' RNA ' molecules which link to specific receptors.

In man, an interest in control gene mutations is not entirely academic. There is always the possibility of discovering chemical agents which might switch on genes which have been switched off. The importance of such agents in the treatment of hereditary disease would, of course, be considerable.

FURTHER READING

Agarwal, K. L., Böchi, H., Caruthers, M. H. *et al.* (1970). Total synthesis of the gene for an alanine transfer ribonucleic acid from yeast. *Nature, Lond.* **227**, 27–34.

Asimov, I. (1962). *The Genetic Code.* New York: Signet Science Library.

Boyer, S. H. (1970). An appraisal of genetic regulation of protein synthesis in higher organisms: 1969. In *Modern Trends in Human Genetics.* Vol. 1. Ed. Emery, A. E. H., pp. 1–41. London: Butterworths.

Dreyfus, J. C. (1969). The application of bacterial genetics to the study of human genetic abnormalities. *Prog. med. Genet.* **6**, 169–200.

Harris, H. (1970). Genetical theory and the ' inborn errors of metabolism ' *Br. med J.* **1**, 321–327.

Jacob, F. and Monod, J. (1961). Genetic regulatory mechanisms in the synthesis of proteins. *J. mol. Biol.* **3**, 318–356.

Ochoa, S. (1964). The chemical basis of heredity—the genetic code. *Bull. N.Y. Acad. Med.* **40**, 387–413.

Sonneborn, T. M. (ed) (1965). *The Control of Human Heredity and Evolution.* London: Macmillan.

Strauss, B. S. (1964). Chemical mutagens and the genetic code. *Prog. med. Genet.* **3**, 1–48.

Temin, H. M. (1972). RNA-directed DNA synthesis. *Sci. Amer.* **226**(1), 25–33.

Watson, J. D. (1970). *Molecular Biology of the Gene,* 2nd ed. New York: Benjamin.

Woods, R. A. (1973). *Biochemical Genetics.* London: Chapman & Hall.

III

Biochemical Genetics

In the previous chapter the biochemistry and mode of action of genes were considered at the molecular level. In this chapter we shall consider the more 'peripheral' biochemical effects of gene action as exemplified in the inborn errors of metabolism, the haemoglobinopathies and the immunoglobulinopathies.

THE INBORN ERRORS OF METABOLISM

At first Garrod, and later Beadle and Tatum, developed the idea that metabolic processes, whether in man or in any other organism, proceed by steps. Each step is controlled by a particular enzyme and this in turn is the product of a particular gene. This is referred to as the ' one gene–one enzyme ' concept, which is illustrated by such conditions as phenylketonuria, alkaptonuria, albinism, and galactosaemia. Phenylketonuria is a particularly distressing condition. Children with this disease are severely mentally retarded, frequently have convulsions, and often have to be institutionalized. In these children a particular enzyme necessary for the conversion of phenylalanine to tyrosine (phenylalanine hydroxylase) is deficient; that is, there is a ' genetic-block ' in the metabolic pathway (fig. 6). As a result, phenylalanine tends to accumulate and some is converted into phenylpyruvic acid which is excreted in the urine. Because of a deficiency of tyrosine, which results from the enzyme block, there is a reduction in melanin formation (fig. 6). Affected children therefore often have blond hair and blue eyes and areas of the brain which are normally pigmented (e.g. the substantia nigra) may also lack pigment.

An obvious method for treating phenylketonuria would be to give the patient the enzyme he lacks but this is not practicable for many reasons. Alternatively it would be expected that if phenylalanine were removed from the diet this might be an effective treatment. In fact this is so. If an affected child is detected early enough, the disease can be prevented by giving a special diet containing little phenylalanine (this is an essential amino acid and therefore cannot be entirely removed from the diet). The condition can be diagnosed by tests which detect phenylpyruvic acid in the urine (ferric chloride test) or excess phenylalanine in the blood (e.g. Guthrie test). Phenyl-ketonuria is not to be confused with hyperphenylalaninaemia. The latter is a benign self-limiting disorder which does not require treatment and is associated with perfectly normal development.

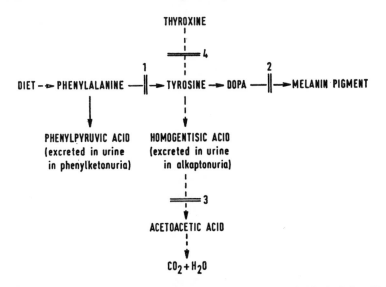

Figure 6. Diagram indicating the sites of 'biochemical blocks' in (1) phenylketonuria, (2) albinism, (3) alkaptonuria and (4) congenital thyroxine deficiency (cretinism).

As we have seen already in alkaptonuria there is a block in the breakdown of homogentisic acid (fig. 6) which therefore accumulates and is excreted in the urine, to which it imparts a dark colour. Dark pigment is also deposited in certain tissues such as the cartilage of the ears and joints. In albinism there is a failure to synthesize the enzyme tyrosinase which is necessary for the formation of melanin pigment from tyrosine (fig. 6). In generalized albinism there is lack of pigment in the skin, hair, the iris, and ocular fundus.

Another condition in man in which a 'genetic-block' has been identified is galactosaemia. This disease also manifests itself in early life and is characterized by vomiting and diarrhoea and failure to thrive. Later complications include severe mental retardation, cataracts, and cirrhosis of the liver. The disease is due to a deficiency of the enzyme necessary for the metabolism of the sugar, galactose (galactose-1-phosphate uridyl transferase). The disease can be prevented by feeding a diet which does not contain galactose (or lactose which, in the body, is broken down into galactose). A number of commercially available milk substitutes can now be obtained which contain neither lactose nor galactose. Early diagnosis and treatment are essential if the severe complications of galactosaemia are to be prevented. The characteristics of a number of inborn errors of metabolism are summarized in table III. Over 120 inborn errors of metabolism are known in which the specific enzyme defect has been identified. These are autosomal recessive (p. 100) or X-linked recessive (p. 104) disorders. The only autosomal dominant disorders (excluding the haemoglobinopathies) in which a specific biochemical disorder has so far been identified are *acute intermittent porphyria, angioneurotic oedema* and possibly *familial hypercholesterolaemia*. In the latter disorder there appears to be a deficiency of a specific protein which regulates cholesterol metabolism. Acute intermittent porphyria is characterised by the excretion of porphyrins in the urine and attacks of abdominal pain and mental aberrations. It is caused by a partial deficiency of uroporphyrinogen I synthetase which is rate-limiting so that even a partial deficiency results in clinical disease when the metabolic pathway is stressed as when barbiturates are taken. Hereditary angioneurotic oedema is a severe, sometimes fatal disorder, characterized by recurrent attacks of oedema of the skin, throat and gut. In this disorder there is a specific deficiency of an inhibitor of the first component of complement. There are two types of deficiency: in one there is a reduction in the total amount of inhibitor, in the other normal amounts of inhibitor are synthesized but with little functional activity. Acute attacks can be treated with infusions of normal fresh-frozen plasma which contains the inhibitor. Attacks can be prevented by aminocaproic acid.

Not all genetically determined disorders are due to a deficiency of an enzyme, but enzymes are proteins and the currently held view of gene action is that genes control the synthesis of proteins. When there is an abnormal gene (mutant gene), a particular protein is either not synthesized at all or, it is synthesized but is defective in some way (p. 22). Normal blood coagulation requires the presence of a particular protein known as antihaemophilic globulin. In haemophilia, there is a deficiency of functionally active antihaemophilic globulin and in this disease there is little difficulty in visualizing the primary cause as being a defect of a specific protein. In fact, in most patients with haemophilia antihaemophilic globulin is synthesized but it is not active: the factor is replaced by a functionally inactive but antigenically similar factor. But in such conditions

Table III. *Characteristics of some inborn errors of metabolism (A.R. & A.D.*
= autosomal recessive or dominant. X.R. & X.D. = X-linked recessive or
dominant)

Disorder	Genetics (usual)	Deficient enzyme or defect	Main clinical features
Acatalasia	A.R.	catalase	? oral sepsis
Adrenogenital syndrome	A.R.	21-hydroxylase in adrenal cortex	virilization
Albinism	A.R.	tyrosinase	1. lack of skin and hair pigment
			2. eye defects
Alkaptonuria	A.R.	homogentisic acid oxidase	
Crigler-Najjar syndrome	A.R.	glucuronyl-transferase in liver	severe jaundice
Cystinuria	A.R.	renal transport defect of cystine	renal stones
Diabetes insipidus	A.D.	deficiency of anti-diuretic hormone	polyuria
	X.R.	kidney unresponsive to anti-diuretic hormone	polyuria
Fibrocystic disease	A.R.	?	1. meconium ileus
			2. intestinal malabsorption
			3. pulmonary disease
Galactosaemia	A.R.	galactose-1-phosphate uridyl transferase	1. mental retardation
			2. cataracts
			3. cirrhosis
Gargoylism:			
1. Hunter's syndrome	X.R.	iduronosulphate sulphatase	1. mental retardation
			2. skeletal abnormalities
			3. hepato-splenomegaly
2. Hurler's syndrome	A.R.	iduronidase	As Hunter's syndrome plus corneal clouding

Disease	Inheritance	Enzyme defect	Clinical features
G6PD deficiency	X.R.	G6PD	induced haemolytic anaemia
Homocystinuria	A.R.	cystathionine synthetase	1. mental retardation 2. dislocation of the lens 3. thrombosis 4. skeletal abnormalities
Lesch-Nyhan syndrome	X.R.	hypoxanthine-guanine phosphoribosyl transferase (HGPRT)	1. mental retardation 2. self mutilation 3. neurological abnormalities
Maple syrup urine disease	A.R.	Branched-chain α-ketoacid decarboxylase	mental retardation
McArdle's syndrome	A.R.	muscle phosphorylase	muscle cramps
Orotic aciduria	A.R.	orotidylate pyrophosphorylase and decarboxylase	megaloblastic anaemia
Phenylketonuria	A.R.	phenylalanine hydroxylase	1. mental retardation 2. fair skin, eczema 3. epilepsy
Tay-Sachs disease (amaurotic idiocy)	A.R.	hexosaminidase-A	1. mental retardation 2. blindness 3. neurological abnormalities
Vitamin-D resistant rickets	X.D.	renal defect in phosphate reabsorption	rickets
Wilson's disease	A.R.	? (abnormal deposition of copper)	1. ataxia 2. cirrhosis

as polydactyly it is at first sight difficult to imagine the primary cause to be an abnormality of a single protein. After all it seems very unlikely that there is a specific protein which determines the formation of extra fingers! It is possible that in ' structural abnormalities ' such as polydactyly, the primary defect involves a more extensive piece of chromosome material than in those conditions which appear more directly related to the effects of a single abnormal or deficient protein. Yet another factor to be considered is that the chain of events from the primary action of the gene to the final outward manifestations of the disorder may be extremely complex because of interactions between various tissues, hormonal influences, and so on.

A good example of just how complex the relationship can be between the primary action of the gene and the ultimate phenotypic expression is provided by the disease of sickle-cell anaemia, one of the haemoglobinopathies. Since the study of the haemoglobinopathies has thrown a great deal of light on the mechanism of gene action this is perhaps a good point to discuss this group of disorders in some detail.

THE HAEMOGLOBINOPATHIES

The haemoglobinopathies are a group of hereditary disorders in which there is an abnormality of the haemoglobin molecule. The haemoglobin molecule is composed of four subunits each of which consists of an iron-containing haem portion and a polypeptide chain (globin). Each haemoglobin molecule usually has two polypeptide chains of one sort and two of another sort. The different sorts of polypeptide chains, by convention are referred to by Greek letters: alpha, α, beta, β, gamma, γ, delta, δ and epsilon, ϵ. There are four main types of normal haemoglobin. The main haemoglobin in adults is referred to as haemoglobin A (Hb A). It has two α and two β polypeptide chains $(\alpha_2\beta_2)$. These two chains have approximately the same length, the α chain containing 141 amino acids and the β chain containing 146 amino acids. Haemoglobin A_2 (Hb A_2), which accounts for about 2 per cent of the haemoglobin present in the blood of an adult, has two α chains and two δ chains $(\alpha_2\delta_2)$, and fetal haemoglobin which is present in the developing fetus but disappears after birth, is composed of two α chains and two γ chains $(\alpha_2\gamma_2)$. Finally there is an embryonic haemoglobin, which is usually present only in early embryonic life and has two α chains and two ϵ chains $(\alpha_2\epsilon_2)$. Five different genes are believed to be responsible for synthesizing the five $(\alpha \beta \gamma \delta \epsilon)$ different peptide chains. The changing patterns in haemoglobin synthesis during development may well reflect differential gene activity. For example, as Hb A gradually replaces fetal haemoglobin, the γ gene is presumably being switched off while at the same time the β gene is being turned on (fig. 7).

Returning now to the story of sickle-cell anaemia, this disease is common in Africa, parts of the Mediterranean area, and India. In certain parts of Africa up to 4 per cent of the population are affected. Affected individuals suffer from a very severe haemolytic anaemia and death often occurs in childhood though occasional individuals may survive into adult life. In 1949 Pauling and his collaborators showed that the haemoglobin in this disease (Hb S)

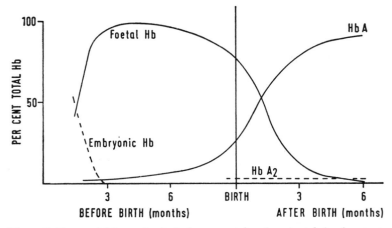

Figure 7. Haemoglobin synthesis during prenatal and postnatal development. (After E. R. Huehns and E. M. Shooter, 1956, *J. med. Genet.* **2**, 52, with permission.)

differs from Hb A with regard to its mobility in an electrical field and they therefore concluded that the globin molecules of Hb A and Hb S must be different. The precise nature of the difference between the globin molecules was identified by Ingram a few years later. He showed that the difference between normal and sickle-cell haemoglobin resided in the β chain and involved only *one* of the 146 amino acids in that chain: at a particular site in the β chain of Hb A (the sixth position from the N-terminus), the amino acid, glutamic acid, was replaced by valine. The molecular 'formulae' for Hb A and Hb S are often written as $\alpha_2^A\beta_2^A$ and $\alpha_2^A\beta_2^S$, respectively, thus indicating that the abnormality in Hb S resides in the β chain. When the amino acid substitution has been located at a particular

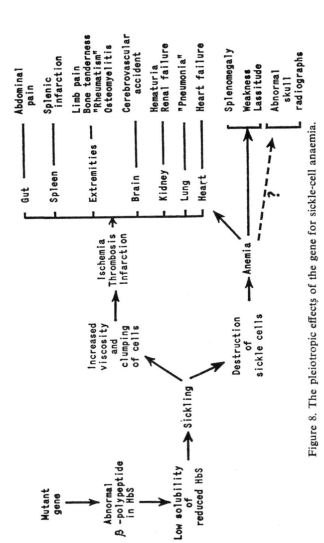

Figure 8. The pleiotropic effects of the gene for sickle-cell anaemia.

site in one of the haemoglobin chains, then a full descriptive formula can be used which indicates the particular substitution. For example, Hb S is $\alpha_2{}^A\beta_2{}^{6Val}$.

The clinical manifestations of sickle-cell anaemia are very numerous and include attacks of abdominal pain, limb pain, ' rheumatism ', cerebral symptoms, kidney failure, ' pneumonia ', heart failure, weakness, and lassitude. All these various manifestations can in fact be traced back to the action of the mutant gene and the substitution of valine for glutamic acid in the β chain of haemoglobin. The abnormal haemoglobin is less soluble than normal haemoglobin and therefore tends to crystallize out resulting in deformation of the red cells which instead of being round become sickle-shaped. The body reacts by destroying these abnormal sickle-cells with the result that a profound anaemia develops with weakness and lassitude. At the same time these abnormal cells tend to clump together and thereby obstruct small arteries resulting in an inadequate oxygen supply to the tissues. If the blood vessels of the kidney are involved, then kidney failure results. If the blood vessels of the heart are involved then heart failure results. The other manifestations of the disease can all be explained similarly (fig. 8). A gene with multiple effects, such as the sickle-cell anaemia gene, is sometimes referred to as being *pleiotropic*.

Sickle-cell anaemia is recessive; that is children with sickle-cell anaemia are homozygous for the mutant gene. The parents are heterozygous and usually normal though their red cells sickle if subjected to low oxygen pressure *in vitro*. Heterozygotes are said to have sickle-cell trait.

Hb C disease is another haemoglobinopathy which also occurs in Africa but in this case individuals homozygous for the mutant gene are much less severely affected than in sickle-cell anaemia. At precisely the same spot in the β polypeptide chain at which the amino acid substitution occurs in Hb S, in Hb C, glutamic acid is replaced by the amino acid lysine ($\alpha_2{}^A\beta_2{}^{6Lys}$). If we assume that the triplet codes in the DNA molecule are CTC for glutamic acid, CAC for valine, and TTC for lysine (see table I, p. 21) then a change in one base from a T to an A could result in the code for valine rather than glutamic acid. Similarly the substitution of a T for a C in the code for glutamic acid would lead to the formation of the code for lysine. Thus the mutation from Hb A to Hb S and Hb A to Hb C could be accounted for by single base substitutions in the same codon. The amino acid substitutions and clinical features of some haemoglobinopathies are given in table IV. A good review of the haemoglobinopathies is to be found in Schwartz (1972).

Table IV. Amino acid substitutions and clinical features of some haemoglobinopathies

Chain	position	from	to	Hb	Clinical
α	58	His	Tyr	M(Boston)	Methaemoglobinaemia
	92	Arg	Leu	Chesapeake	Hb has increased O_2 affinity, Polycythaemia
	92	Arg	Gln	J(Cape Town)	,,
β	6	Glu	Val	S	Haemolytic anaemia
	6	Glu	Lys	C	,,
	63	His	Arg	Zurich	Drug induced haemolysis
	92	His	Tyr	M(Hyde Park)	Methaemoglobinaemia
	98	Val	Gly	Nottingham	Haemolytic anaemia
	102	Asp	Thr	Kansas	Hb has reduced O_2 affinity, Cyanosis
	103	Phe	Leu	Heathrow	Hb has increased O_2 affinity, Polycythaemia
γ	121	Glu	Lys	F(Hull)	—
δ	22	Ala	Glu	Flatbush	—

Amino acids are abbreviated: Ala, alanine; Arg, arginine; Asp, aspartic acid; Gln, glutamine; Glu, glutamic acid; His, histidine; Leu, leucine; Lys, lysine; Phe, phenylalanine; Thr, threonine; Tyr, tyrosine; Val, valine.

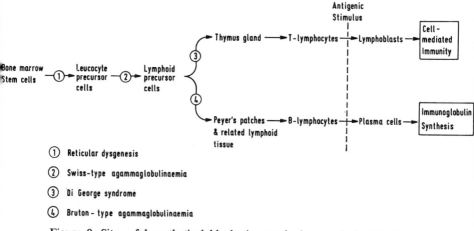

① Reticular dysgenesis

② Swiss-type agammaglobulinaemia

③ Di George syndrome

④ Bruton - type agammaglobulinaemia

Figure 9. Sites of hypothetical blocks in certain immunological deficiency
diseases.

Haemoglobinopathies have also been recognized where the α
chain or β chain is longer than normal as in Hb Constant Spring
and Hb Tak respectively. It is believed that the normal m-RNA
for Hb chains is longer than that needed to code for the actual
protein and the haemoglobinopathies with elongated chains may
therefore be the result of *termination* mutations.

In order to include such hereditary conditions as sickle-cell
anaemia and the other haemoglobinopathies, the ' one gene-one
enzyme' concept is best rephrased as '*one gene–one polypeptide*'.
The gene is that unit which specifies the amino acid sequence of one
polypeptide and is made up of many codons. The term *cistron* is
sometimes used for the smallest unit of genetic material which
directs the synthesis of a specific polypeptide.

So far we have discussed the group of haemoglobinopathies
characterized by structural alterations in one of the globin peptide
chains. There is, however, another group of haemoglobinopathies
in which there is a defect in the *rate of synthesis* of globin chains.
This second group constitutes the so-called thalassaemia syndromes
which are characterized either by a defect in the synthesis of α-
chains (α-thalassaemias) or of β-chains (β-thalassaemias). In the
case of α-thalassaemia recent research indicates that this disorder
is due to an actual *deletion* of the α-chain of haemoglobin gene. In α-
thalassaemia the homozygote dies *in utero*, in β-thalassaemia the
homozygote has a severe anaemia. In these conditions the heterozygote may or may not have clinical symptoms. The thalassaemias are
a very heterogeneous group of disorders, and their investigation is

helping us to understand more of the gene control of haemoglobin synthesis.

THE IMMUNOGLOBULINOPATHIES

The immunoglobulins are a class of serum proteins which in some ways resemble the haemoglobins. Their structure and function is gradually being understood and their genetic significance appreciated.

The immune system of man may be conveniently considered under two headings: the immunoglobulin-producing function and cellular immunity. It is believed that during development a lymphoid precursor cell may take one of two alternative pathways. The first involves the formation of the thymus gland and differentiation into small lymphocytes which are found in the cortical regions of the lymph nodes and in the spleen, and are responsible for cellular immunity (transplantation immunity or homograft rejection and delayed hypersensitivity). Alternatively the precursor cells may differentiate into plasma cells which are found in the germinal centres of the lymph nodes as well as in Peyer's patches in the intestine, and are responsible for the synthesis of immunoglobulins (fig. 9). This idea provides a working model for understanding the nature of certain immunological deficiency diseases in man.

The immunoglobulins (Ig) are serum proteins which act as antibodies, being important in the body's defence mechanisms against infection. Papaine, a proteolytic enzyme, splits the immunoglobulin molecule into three fragments which can be separated by chromatography. Two of the fragments are similar each containing an antibody site capable of combining with a specific antigen and therefore referred to as *Fab* (= Fragment—antigen—binding). The third fragment has no antibody activity but because it can be crystallized it is referred to as *Fc* (= Fragment—crystallizable). The immunoglobulin molecule is made up of four polypeptide chains: two 'light' (L) and two 'heavy' (H), held together by disulphide bonds. Each *Fab* is composed of L-chains and parts of the H-chains, whereas *Fc* is composed only of parts of the H-chains. A proposed structure of the immunoglobulin molecule is given in figure 10. The L-chains can be further subdivided into kappa (κ) and lambda (λ) types. Some recent studies suggest that the kappa and lambda L-chains are each synthesized by two separate genes and therefore appear to be an exception to the rule of 'one gene–one polypeptide chain'.

There are five major classes of immunoglobulins designated as IgG, IgM, IgA, IgD and IgE (Table V). The two types of L-chains are common to all five classes of immunoglobulins, but the H-

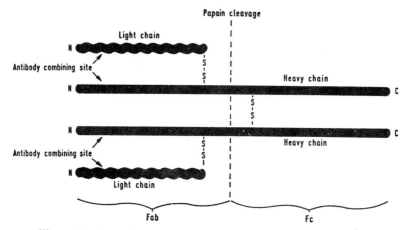

Figure 10. A proposed structure of the immunoglobulin molecule.

chains are different in each class, i.e. IgG, IgM, IgA, IgD and IgE heavy chains are designated respectively as γ, μ, α, δ and ϵ. Thus the molecular formula for IgG is $\gamma_2\kappa_2\gamma_2\lambda_2$ and for IgM is $\mu_2\kappa_2\mu_2\lambda_2$ etc.

There is little synthesis of immunoglobulin by the fetus but adult levels are attained by the end of the first year.

The five classes of immunoglobulins occur in all normal individuals but genetically determined variants of these classes have also been identified. These are the *Gm* system associated with the H-chain of IgG, the *Am* system associated with the H-chain of

Table V. *Classes of human immunoglobulins*

Class	Mol. wt.	Serum concentration (mg/ml)	Antibody activity	Placental transfer
IgG	150,000	12·0	to bacteria and viruses (most antibodies)	+
IgM	900,000	1·0	to protein antigens (some blood groups and bacteria)	—
IgA	160,000+	2·5	in external secretions (local immunity)	? +
IgD	180,000	0·03	?	—
IgE	200,000	trace	in allergic reactions	—

Table VI. *Some immunological deficiency diseases* (A.R. = autosomal recessive; X.R. = X-linked recessive)

Disorder	*Site of defect	Thymus gland	Lymphocytes	Cell-mediated immunity	Plasma cells	Ig Synthesis	Genetics	Treatment
Reticular dysgenesis (absence of leucocytes)	1	absent	→	→	→	→	?A.R.	—
Swiss-type agammaglobulinaemia	2	vestigeal	→	→	→	→	A.R.	transplantation of fetal thymus and compatible bone marrow cells
DiGeorge syndrome	3	absent (parathyroids absent as well)	+	→	+	N	—	? transplantation of fetal thymus
Bruton-type agammaglobulinaemia	4	+	+	N	→	→	X.R.	Ig injections and antibiotics

* possible site of defect—see figure 9.

IgA, the *Inv* system associated with the kappa L-chain and the *Oz* associated with the lambda L-chain. The Gm and Am groups are controlled by multiple allelles at a single autosomal locus (or at several closely linked loci) as are the Inv groups. The Gm and Inv systems are independent of each other and are polymorphic (p. 167), the frequencies of the various alleles of the Gm and Inv loci being different in various racial groups. So far no genetic variants have been identified with the H-chains of IgM or IgD though they no doubt exist.

The manifestations of at least some of the immunological deficiency diseases of man (table VI) can best be understood by assuming that defects have occurred at specific points in the immune system as given in figure 9 (if only as an aide-mémoire). However it should be emphasized that several rare immunological deficiency diseases do not fit into this simplified scheme. Whenever cellular immunity is depressed this is associated with prolonged survival of skin homografts and susceptibility to virus infections. Whenever Ig synthesis is depressed this is associated with reduced resistance to bacterial infections which may lead to death in infancy as in Swiss-type agammaglobulinaemia. Interestingly, though the Gm and Inv groups are definitely autosomal and therefore the IgG H-chains and the kappa L-chains are synthesized by autosomal genes, Bruton-type agammaglobulinaemia is an X-linked recessive trait. Perhaps this disorder is due to a mutation of a particular locus on the X-chromosome which normally acts as a regulator gene for the autosomal loci responsible for Ig synthesis.

Certain hereditary disorders are known in which there is a deficiency in only one or two of the immunoglobulin groups, the remainder being normal or elevated. These latter conditions are referred to as the *dysgammaglobulinaemias*. Affected individuals are unduly susceptible to respiratory tract infections. There are also the *hypogammaglobulinaemias* in which Ig levels are reduced but not absent. The dysgammaglobulinaemias and the hypogammaglobulinaemias are heterogeneous and include cases of both genetic and environmental origin.

There are also a number of hereditary syndromes in which Ig abnormalities are a feature. These include the ataxia-telangiectasia syndrome (an autosomal recessive) in which there is cerebellar ataxia, oculocutaneous telangiectasia (dilated blood capillaries) and a susceptibility to sinus and pulmonary infections, the thymus is hypoplastic and serum levels of IgA are reduced. Another syndrome, the Wiskott-Aldrich syndrome (X-linked recessive) is associated with thrombocytopaenia, eczema, diarrhoea and recurrent infections. IgM levels are usually low and affected boys usually die in childhood. This disorder has recently been treated with transplantation of compatible bone marrow cells. Finally, in myotonic dystrophy (an inherited muscle disease) there is evidence of increased catabolism of IgG.

The precise cause of any of the immunoglobulinopathies is at present unknown. They present a challenge both to the immunochemist interested in aetiology and to the physician presented with the problem of finding an effective treatment.

TRANSPLANTATION GENETICS

In recent years considerable interest has developed in the possibilities of replacing diseased organs by healthy ones removed either from healthy living donors or from cadavers. Except for corneal and bone grafts, the success of such transplants depends on the degree of antigenic similarity between the donor and recipient. The closer the similarity, the greater the likelihood that the transplanted organ or tissue (homograft) will be accepted rather than rejected. Homograft rejection does not occur in identical twins or in certain nonidentical twins where there has been mixing of the placental circulations before birth (p. 78). In all other instances the donor and recipient have to be matched not only for the ABO blood groups but also for what are referred to as the HL-A (histo-compatibility locus-A) antigens, which are carried on various tissues including leucocytes. The leucocyte antigens so far defined are inherited as codominant traits (p. 104) so that whenever a gene is present its appropriate antigen is demonstrable. As a general rule a recipient will reject a graft from any person who has antigens which the recipient lacks. Thus, by analogy with the ABO red cell system a person of group A is likely to accept a graft from an individual of group A but not from someone of group B or AB, but a person of group AB is likely to accept grafts from individuals who are group A, B or AB. The same principle holds true for the HL-A antigens.

The histocompatibility (antigenic similarity) of donor and recipient may be assessed by methods which depend on *matching* the donor and recipient by serological *tissue typing*. Matching may also be carried out by the mixed lymphocyte culture (MLC) test. In the MLC test, lymphocytes from donor and recipient are mixed *in vitro*. Here the lymphocyte is used both as a responding cell (reacting to foreign antigens by enlargement, DNA synthesis and division) and as a stimulating cell (carrying the foreign antigens). The extent of the response of the lymphocytes in culture is used to assess the amount of antigenic disparity between two individuals. With regard to tissue typing, suitable antisera are used to identify antigens on donor and recipient tissues. Here lymphocyte agglutination or cytotoxicity may be used as indicators of antigen-antibody reactions. In the case of the lymphocyte cytotoxicity test, lymphocytes are incubated with each of many antisera and trypan blue stain, which only stains dead cells, is added later. If the lymphocytes carry an antigen to which an antibody is present in a particular serum then the cells will be killed and will appear blue stained. By matching with the MLC test with the object of minimizing HL-A disparity, or by typing for HL-A antigens, a prospective donor and recipient are matched as closely as possible.

The HL-A system consists of a group of closely linked loci: two major loci called LA (or I) and Four (or II) as well as other loci concerned with immune response (Ir locus) and reactivity in mixed lymphocytic culture (MLC locus). So far 14 alleles at the LA locus and 27 alleles at the Four locus have been identified. These various alleles can be combined to produce more than 70,000 different genotypes. Each individual has two LA and two Four genes, and a parent will always share one of its two HL-A chromosomes with any of its children. Furthermore, any individual will have a 25 per cent chance of having identical antigens with a sib since there are only four possible combinations of the two paternal HL-A chromosomes (say A and B) with the two maternal HL-A chromosomes (say C and D), i.e. AC, AD, BC, and BD. Thus the sibs of a particular recipient are more likely to be antigenically similar to him than either of his parents, and the latter more than an unrelated person. For this reason a brother or sister is frequently selected as a donor. At the same time the recipients immune mechanisms are suppressed by immunosuppressive drugs (e.g. azathioprine, steroids, antilymphocytic serum). In recent series with antigenic matching and immunosuppressive therapy, the three year survival rate of live-donor renal transplants has exceeded 60 per cent. There is a suggestion that a graft is more likely to be accepted if donor and recipient are particularly matched for the second HL-A sublocus, the reason for which is not yet clear. As knowledge of tissue typing increases no doubt greater success will be achieved not only with renal transplants but possibly also with other tissues.

FURTHER READING

Bach, F. H. (1970). Transplantation: pairing of donor and recipient. *Science, N.Y.* **168**, 1170–1179.
Bradley, J. (1974) Immunoglobulins—a review. *J. med. Genet.* **11**, 80-90.

Brock, D. J. H. & Mayo, O. (1972). Editors. *The Biochemical Genetics of Man*. London & New York: Academic Press.

Franglen, G. (1970). Immune globulin deficiencies. *Br. J. hosp. Med.* **3**, 651–660.

Harris, R. (1975). *The Principles of Human Biochemical Genetics*. 2nd ed. Amsterdam: North Holland.

Harris, R. (1969). Evolution of cellular immunity and the genetics of human organ transplantation. In *Selected Topics in Medical Genetics*. Ed. Clarke, C. A., pp. 135–158. Oxford University Press.

Harris, R. (1975). Genetics and immunology in human leukaemia. In *Modern Trends in Human Genetics*. Vol. 2. Ed. Emery, A. E. H. pp. 138-176. London: Butterworths.

Holborow, E. J. (1973). 2nd edit. *An ABC of Modern Immunology*. London: Lancet.

Kissmeyer-Nielsen, F., Jørgensen, F. & Lamm, L. U. (1972). The HL-A system in clinical medicine. *Hopkins med. J.* **131**, 385–400.

Lehmann, H. & Carrell, R. W. (1969). Variations in the structure of human haemoglobin. *Br. med. Bull.* **25**(1), 14–23.

Nathan, D. G. (1972). Thalassaemia. *New Engl. J. Med.* **286**, 586–594.

Raeburn, J. A. (1975). Genetic defects of leucocyte function. In *Modern Trends in Human Genetics*. Vol. 2. Ed. Emery, A. E. H. pp. 177-203. London: Butterworths.

Rosen, F. S., *et al.* (1966). The gamma globulins. *New Engl. J. Med.* **275**, (series of articles in numbers 9–15; Sept. 1–Oct. 13).

Schimke, R. N. & Kirkpatrick, C. H. (1970). Genetic disorders of gamma-globulin synthesis. In *Modern Trends in Human Genetics*. Vol. 1. Ed. Emery, A. E. H. pp. 68–103. London: Butterworths.

Schwartz, E. (1972). Haemoglobinopathies of clinical importance. *Ped. Clin. N. Amer.* **19**, 889–905.

Sherwood, L. M., Parris, E. E. & Ranney, H. M. (1970). Clinically important variants of human haemoglobin. *New Engl. J. Med.* **282**, 144–152.

Turk, J. L. (1969). *Immunology in Clinical Medicine*. London: Heinemann.

Wetherall, D. J. (1969). The genetics of the thalassaemias. *Br. med. Bull.* **25**(1), 24–29.

Weir, D. M. (1970). *Immunology for Undergraduates*. Edinburgh: Livingstone.

Woodrow, J. C. (1969). Some aspects of immunogenetics. In *Selected Topics in Medical Genetics*. Ed. Clarke, C. A., pp. 159–182. Oxford University Press.

IV

Chromosomes and Chromosomal Abnormalities

CHROMOSOME STRUCTURE AND NUMBER

Chromosomes can be made visible by special staining techniques only during the period when the nucleus is dividing. This is because the chromosomes at this time are contracted, thicker, and take up stains better than in the resting nucleus. Each chromosome is not uniform in width throughout its length but has a nipped-in portion referred to as the *centromere*. The exact structure of the centromere is a subject of some controversy but it is known to be responsible for the movement of the chromosomes at nuclear division. The centromere is located near the centre of some chromosomes which are then referred to as metacentric chromosomes, and near the end of others which are referred to as acrocentric chomosomes. When the centromere is not exactly in the centre, the chromosome is divided into two arms of unequal length—a long arm and a short arm.

Individual chromosomes differ not only in the position of the centromere but also in their total length. In many cases it is therefore possible to identify individual chromosomes using these two criteria.

Each nucleus in a somatic cell contains two sets of chromosomes, the members of a pair of chromosomes being referred to as homologues. One member of a pair of *homologous chromosomes* is derived from one parent and the other member of the pair from the other parent.

The number of chromosomes is halved when the gametes are formed. Nuclei in the cells of the body thus contain twice as many chromosomes as nuclei in the gametes (sex cells): with regard to the number of chromosomes the somatic cells are said to be *diploid* whereas those of the gametes are said to be *haploid*.

The number of chromosomes in different organisms varies considerably but is constant for any particular species. In certain ferns there are as many as 500 chromosomes within a single nucleus, and one small crustacean is estimated to have somewhere between 1500 and 1600 chromosomes per nucleus. At the other extreme, one intestinal worm is known in which the diploid number of chromosomes is only two.

A few years ago it was thought that the number of chromosomes might be of some help in determining the relationship between various groups of primates. But investigations soon showed that the situation was much more complicated. Whereas the marmoset and certain monkeys resemble man in having 46 chromosomes, higher primates more closely related to man, such as the gorilla, chimpanzee, and orangutan, have 48 chromosomes. The relationships between various groups of animals must depend on the genes carried by the chromosomes more than on the number of chromosomes.

There are two types of chromosomes, those concerned with sex determination which are referred to as the *sex chromosomes* and the remainder which are referred to as the *autosomes*. The credit for being the first investigator to identify sex chromosomes goes to Henking. In 1891 Henking, a German cytologist, noticed that during spermatogenesis in certain insects a particular chromosome migrated undivided to one end of the dividing nucleus. In this way one sperm came to possess this chromosome while the other did not. Because of uncertainty as to its exact nature this chromosome was referred to as the ' X ' chromosome. Later on when this chromosome was shown to be the sex-determining chromosome, the letter X was retained to designate the sex chromosome. In the particular insects studied by Henking the male has only one sex chromosome and this is represented as XO, whereas the female has two sex chromosomes which are represented as XX. But in man and most animals, both the male and the female have two sex chromosomes. In the female they are the same (i.e., XX) but in the male one sex chromosome is the same as the female (i.e. an X chromosome) while the other is smaller and is not found in the female. It is referred to as the Y chromosome. The male is therefore said to have an XY sex chromosome constitution. In the female each ovum carries either of the X chromosomes but in the male each sperm carries either an X or a Y chromosome. Since there is about an equal chance of either an X-bearing sperm or a Y-bearing sperm fertilizing an egg this explains why the number of male births is approximately (but not exactly) the same as the number of female births:

Male gametes

	X	Y
X	XX	XY
X	XX	XY

Female gametes

MITOSIS

After birth brain cells divide rarely, if at all, whereas other cells, such as those of the bone marrow or those in the deeper layers of the skin, continue to divide throughout life. A skin cell divides about once every three or four days. This means that during a person's lifetime such a cell will have divided nearly 10,000 times! This leaves a lot of room for error, yet in fact the process is extremely well regulated for mistakes during nuclear division seem to occur very rarely. The process of nuclear division is referred to as *mitosis*. During mitosis each chromosome divides in two and so the number of chromosomes per nucleus remains unchanged. This is the essential feature of mitosis.

Mitosis can be divided into stages but it must be emphasized that the whole process is really a continuous one and does not really take place in separate stages. It is merely divided into stages for the convenience of description (fig. 11).

Interphase: this is the resting stage when the cell is not dividing and the chromosomes are difficult to visualize. There is evidence that towards the end of this stage each chromosome divides longitudinally into two daughter chromosomes, or chromatids, though they remain attached to each other at the centromere.

Prophase: the chromosomes can now be clearly recognized because they are contracted and thus much thicker and take up stains more readily.

Metaphase: the nuclear membrane disappears and the chromosomes become orientated in the centre of the nucleus on the so-called equatorial plate. At the same time the spindle forms. This structure is responsible for the movement of the chromosomes during mitosis. It is at this stage that the chromosomes are best seen; each resembles the letter ' X ' in shape because the centromere does not divide until the next stage.

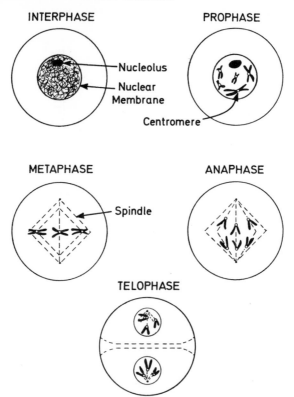

Figure 11. Stages of mitosis.

Anaphase: the centromere of each chromosome now divides into two. The two chromatids move apart to opposite ends of the spindle.

Telophase: the daughter chromosomes have separated completely and the two groups of daughter chromosomes each become invested in a nuclear membrane. The two new cells now separate and their nuclei enter the interphase stage once more.

MEIOSIS

Meiosis is the process of nuclear division which occurs when the gametes are formed. During meiosis the number of chromosomes is halved, each gamete receiving either of a pair of homologous chromosomes but rarely both. Meiosis takes place in two steps, each of which has a prophase, metaphase, anaphase, and telophase stage as in mitosis (fig. 12). In the first step, called meiosis I, the prophase stage is very long. The chromosomes enter this stage already divided longitudinally into two chromatids though the centromeres do not divide until later. During prophase of meiosis I, homologous chromosomes pair and an exchange of parts between

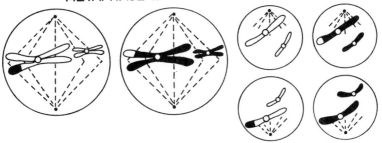

Figure 12. Stages of meiosis.

the chromatids of homologous chromosomes may occur. This process is referred to as crossing-over, the significance of which will be referred to later. The members of each pair of homologous chromosomes migrate to opposite ends of the dividing nucleus, so that each daughter nucleus receives only one member of each pair.

The second step is called meiosis II during which the centromeres divide and the chromatids migrate into separate nuclei. Meiosis II therefore resembles mitosis except that each nucleus contains only the haploid number of chromosomes.

With the formation of the egg and sperm (gametogenesis), the number of chromosomes is halved so that the zygote (which results from the union of egg and sperm) still has the same number of chromosomes as either parent. It is now possible to see how Mendelian inheritance works: at meiosis the number of chromosomes is halved and each gamete receives one or the other of each pair of homologous chromosomes (and consequently the genes it carries).

Homologous chromosomes look alike and at identical positions on each chromosome are genes determining the same characteristic. But these genes, though determining the same characteristic, may not be identical. For example, situated on the X chromosome is a gene which produces a protein (antihaemophilic globulin) necessary for normal blood clotting. In the disease haemophilia the gene fails to produce this protein. A female who carries this disease has the normal gene on one of her X chromosomes and the abnormal (= mutant) gene on her other X chromosome. According to the chromosome theory of inheritance, at meiosis each gamete receives either one of a pair of homologous chromosomes. The female carrier of haemophilia therefore transmits to any particular offspring either the X chromosome bearing the normal gene or the X chromosome bearing the mutant (haemophilia) gene. On the average half her sons will therefore be affected and half will be normal (see p. 107).

GENETIC LINKAGE

As a result of the phenomenon of crossing-over during meiosis there is exchange of chromosomal material between homologous chromosomes. This leads to recombinations of genes, that is, if two genes were originally located on the same chromosome of a particular chromosome pair, crossing-over would result in their becoming separated. Alternatively, if the two genes were originally located on different chromosomes of a particular chromosome pair, crossing-over would result in the two genes being brought together on the same chromosome. When two different genes are located on the same chromosome pair they are said to be *linked*. Clearly crossing-over is more likely to occur between genes which are far apart; conversely, the closer two genes are on any particular chromosome the less likelihood there is that crossing-over will occur. In other words, we can assess the relative distances between genes on any particular chromosome by determining the frequency with which crossing-over occurs between these genes. Distances between genes are measured in map units: one map unit being equal to 1 per cent of crossing-over. Thus, if 5 per cent of the offspring of informative matings are of the recombinant type (i.e. the result of crossing-over) then the two gene loci are said to be about 5 map units apart. Values for the percentage recombination are often greater in females than in males, the reason for which is not clear.

In the 1930s Thomas Hunt Morgan and Calvin Bridges and their colleagues at Columbia University, carried out extensive breeding experiments using the fruit fly *Drosophila*. By careful and pains-taking work they were able to localize certain genes to particular sites on specific chromosomes. By determining the frequency of re-combinant types among the progeny from various crosses they were able to draw up maps of the chromosomes of *Drosophila melano-gaster* indicating the exact positions on each of its four pairs of chromosomes of nearly 100 different genes.

It has also been possible to construct linkage maps for the corn plant, mouse, *Neurospora,* and certain microorganisms. In man a linkage map with the groupings of genes on particular chromo-somes is becoming possible but progress until recently has been slow. The reason is that in the past we had to rely on finding infor-mative matings which have occurred by chance. These are usually rare. For example, in order to determine the relative positions on the X chromosome of the genes for X-linked Duchenne muscular dystrophy (p. 108) and haemophilia it would be necessary to study families in which both diseases occurred together. But these diseases are rare and the chances of their occurring in the same family are extremely small. In fact not one such family has ever been described. In genetic linkage studies in man we have to rely on the information we can obtain by studying the segregation of so-called ' marker ' genes in families with a particular hereditary disorder.

Marker genes are genes which are so frequent in the general population that there is a very good chance they will be present in the family being studied. The autosomal marker traits include the blood groups, certain serum proteins (haptoglobins, transferrins, and so-called Gm proteins), and the ability to taste phenylthiocarbamide

(PTC). The X-linked marker traits include colour blindness, the Xg blood group, Xm serum factor and in certain populations, glucose-6-phosphate dehydrogenase deficiency (G6PD). Pedigree studies have demonstrated linkage between such loci as the ABO blood-group and a rare disorder in which the nails are deformed and the patellae are deficient (nail-patella syndrome); the Lutheran blood-group and ' secretor ' which controls the secretion of certain blood-group substances in the saliva and other body fluids; the rhesus blood-group and one form of elliptocytosis, a haematological condition in which the red cells are oval in shape; and the Duffy blood-group and one form of congenital cataract.

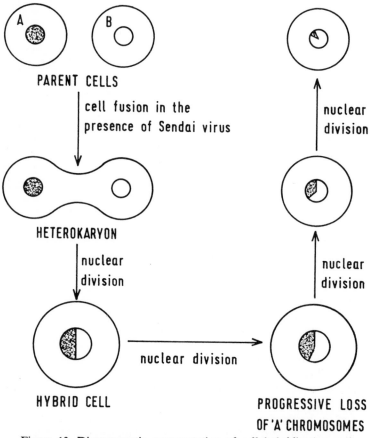

Figure 13. Diagrammatic representation of cell hybridization and subsequent selective loss of chromosomes from the hybrid cells.

With regard to the X chromosome it appears that the loci for phosphoglycerate kinase, Lesch-Nyhan syndrome (p. 31) G6PD, haemophilia A, colour vision, Becker muscular dystrophy (p. 215) and the Xm serum factor are clustered on the long arm. This cluster is located some distance from the Xg blood group locus which is probably situated toward the end of the short arm of the X chromosome. There is evidence that the Xg locus is within measurable distance of the genes for X-linked ichthyosis vulgaris, a condition characterized by a dry scaly and thickened skin, ocular albinism, retinoschisis (one form of retinal detachment), angiokeratoma, a skin condition, and X-linked mental retardation with or without hydrocephalus.

So far we have been discussing gene localization as determined by pedigree analysis and the segregation of different traits within a family, but other approaches to this problem are also possible. Genes may be localized by studying patients with a chromosome deletion (p. 64) for the presence of rare recessive disorders which may be 'uncovered' because of the loss of the normal allele on the deleted chromosome or from the segregation of a marker in a family with a deleted chromosome. In this way, for example, red cell acid phosphatase has been localized to the short arm of chromosome 2. Secondly genes may be localized by the abnormal segregation of a marker trait or disorder in a family with a chromosome abnormality. In this way the gene for the Duffy blood group (and therefore for a particular type of congenital cataract) was localized to chromosome 1. Yet another approach to the problem is to study possible dosage effects in individuals who are trisomic (p. 61) for a particular chromosome. In this way it has been suggested, but not proven, that the gene for superoxide dismutase is on chromosome 21. Finally somatic-cell genetics is proving particularly valuable in genetic linkage studies (Ruddle, 1973). By this technique cells from two different species are fused (using a virus) then cultured, and the resulting changes in the chromosome constitution of the cell-hybrid studied along with concomitant enzyme changes (Fig. 13). For example, mouse cells unable to synthesize thymidine kinase, have been fused with human cells which can synthesize this enzyme. After several generations all the human chromosomes were lost from the hybrid with the exception of one (chromosome 17) yet the hybrid retained the ability to synthesize thymidine kinase thus indicating that the gene for this particular enzyme is located on chromosome 17. Some linkages which have been established by these various techniques are summarized in table VII. A tentative map of chromosome 1 is shown in figure 14.

Table VII. *Gene Localization on the autosomes.*

The loci within linkage groups are not necessarily arranged in order

A *Assigned groups*

Chromosome	Linkage group
1	Un-1 : PGD : PPH : Rh : PGM_1 : Amy_1 : AK_2 :
	El Amy_2
	Cae : Fy : PepC : UDGP
	AOD
2	AcP : Db : MNS : Tys
6	HL-A : IPO(B) : MDH : PGM_3
7	MPI : PK_3
10	GOT : HK
11	LDH(A) : ESA_4
12	LDH(B) : Pep(B)
14	NPR
16	LCAT : Hp : APT
17	TK
18	PepA
19	PHI
21	IPO(A) : SD

B *Unassigned groups*

ABO : NP : AK
Dm : Se : Lu
Pelger Huet : MD
$Hb\beta$: $Hb\delta$: $Hb\gamma$
Alb : Gc
E_1 : Tf
Am : Gm : Pi
PTC : Kell
GPT : EP

Key

AcP = red cell acid phosphatase	Db = Dombrock blood group
ADA = adenosine deaminase	Dm = myotonic dystrophy
AK = adenylate kinase	E = pseudocholinesterase
Alb = albumin variant	El = elliptocytosis
Am = immunoglobulin	EP = epidermolysis (one type)
Amy_1	ESA = esterase A
&	Fy = Duffy blood group
Amy_2 = salivary and pancreatic amylase	Gc = Gc serum protein
	Gm = immunoglobulin
AOD = auriculo-osteodysplasia	GOT = glutamic oxaloacetic trans-
APT = adenosine phosphoribosyltransferase	aminase
	GPT = glutamic pyruvic trans-
Cae = congenital cataract (' zonular ')	aminase
	HK = hexokinase

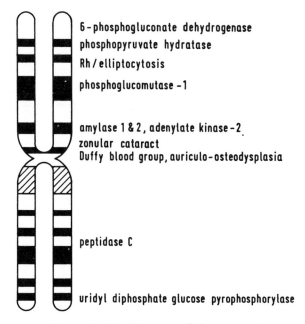

6-phosphogluconate dehydrogenase
phosphopyruvate hydratase
Rh / elliptocytosis

phosphoglucomutase -1

amylase 1 & 2, adenylate kinase -2
zonular cataract
Duffy blood group, auriculo-osteodysplasia

peptidase C

uridyl diphosphate glucose pyrophosphorylase

Figure 14. A tentative map of chromosome 1.

A knowledge of the localization and arrangement of gene loci on chromosomes is not just of academic interest. The hope is that such information will prove valuable in the detection of heterozygous carriers and preclinical cases of certain genetic disorders and perhaps also in antenatal diagnosis.

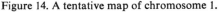

HL-A = histocompatibility locus
Hp   = haptoglobin
IPO = indophenoloxidase
LDH = lactate dehydrogenase
Lu   = Lutheran blood group
MD = muscular dystrophy (one type)
MDH = malate dehydrogenase
MNS = MNS blood group
MPI = mannose phosphate isomerase
Np   = nail-patella syndrome
NPR = nucleoside phosphorylase
Pep = peptidase
PGD = phosphogluconate dehydrogenase

PGM = phosphoglucomutase
PHI   = phosphohexose isomerase
Pi   = α-antitrypsin
PK_3 = pyruvate kinase (leucocyte)
PPH = phosphopyruvate hydratase
PTC = tasting
Rh   = rhesus blood group
Se   = secretor status
SD   = superoxide dismutase
Tf   = transferrin
Tk   = thymidine kinase
Tys   = sclerotylosis
UDGP = uridyl diphosphate glucose pyrophosphorylase
Un   = ' uncoiler '

METHODS OF HUMAN CYTOGENETICS

Even before the beginning of the present century many investigators had attempted to determine the number of chromosomes in man but such investigations were hampered by poor technique. Nevertheless in 1912 Winiwater came very close to the right answer when he claimed that there were 47 chromosomes in man. In the early 1920s Painter expressed the belief that there were 48 chromosomes and this was generally accepted for over 30 years until work of Tjio and Levan in 1956 showed that this was not so. These investigators introduced greatly improved methods for the study of chromosomes which enabled them to demonstrate quite clearly that the diploid number of chromosomes in man was 46. The methods they used, with certain modifications, are now universally employed in all cytogenetic laboratories (fig. 15).

A variety of tissues has been used in studying human chromosomes but most commonly specimens of skin, bone marrow, or peripheral blood are used. In the case of blood, the leucocytes are separated off and added to a small volume of nutrient medium containing phytohaemagglutinin. The addition of phytohaemagglutinin, a substance extracted from the French bean (*Phaseolus vulgaris*); is very important because it stimulates the leucocytes to divide. The cells are cultured under sterile conditions at body temperature (37°C) for about three days. During this time the cells divide and then a small amount of colchicine is added to each culture. Colchicine is a complex organic compound which is extracted from the autumn crocus and had been used for several years before the advent of human cytogenetics in the treatment of gout. Colchicine has the unique property of preventing the formation of the spindle and stops mitosis at the stage of metaphase when the chromosomes are maximally contracted and most clearly defined. After an hour or so a hypotonic saline solution is added. This makes the cells swell and has the effect of spreading the chromosomes which otherwise would remain clumped together and make the accurate counting of chromosomes very difficult.

The next step is to photograph the resulting chromosome 'spread' with the aid of a higher-power microscope with a camera attachment (fig. 16). Later the individual chromosomes are cut out from the photograph, arranged in pairs and in decreasing order of size and numbered from 1 to 22 with the two sex chromosomes indicated separately (fig. 17). Until recently, because it was not possible to distinguish between individual chromosomes, many investigators divided them into seven groups A to G depending on size and the

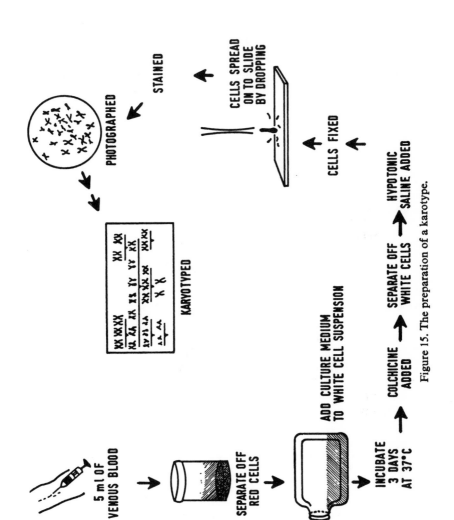

Figure 15. The preparation of a karotype.

position of the centromere. The resulting arrangement of the chromosomes is referred to as the *karyotype*.

CHROMOSOME IDENTIFICATION

The technique of *autoradiography* has been used in an attempt to improve on the identification of individual chromosomes. In this technique cultures are exposed to radioactive thymidine and then after a given time all cell divisions are stopped. Those chromosomes

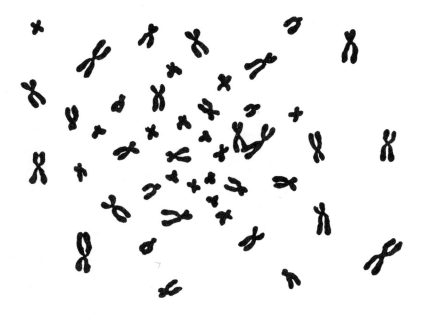

Figure 16. A photomicrograph of a chromosome ' spread '. Each chromosome consists of two chromatids joined at the centromere (magnification about 1500 ×).

which are found to be heavily labelled are those which have incorporated the radioactive thymidine, and have therefore replicated during the period of exposure to radioactive thymidine. Those chromosomes which are not labelled are those which had replicated *before* exposure to radioactive thymidine.

The results of experiments using this technique have shown that not all the chromosomes replicate synchronously. Some replicate

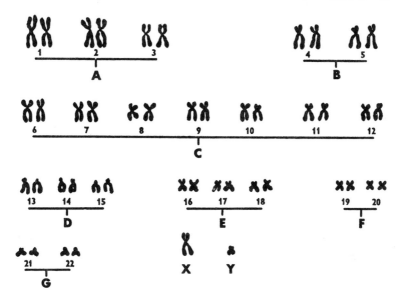

Figure 17. Karyotype of a normal male. Appearance with conventional staining.

later than others. The X chromosome which is to become inactivated (p. 86) can be identified by autoradiography as a late-replicating chromosome of group C size. This is a laborious technique and has now been superseded by improved staining techniques which permit the precise identification of each individual chromosome. There are essentially four different staining techniques: the quinacrine fluorescence or Q method whereby certain chromosome bands appear as fluorescent regions with fluorescent microscopy, various Giemsa or G methods whereby these same bands appear as dark staining regions, the so-called ' reverse ' or R banding method, and special techniques for staining the centromeric region or C methods. The banding patterns of each chromosome are specific and make it possible to identify each individual chromosome (fig. 18). The quinacrine fluorescent technique has also revealed a number of regions in the chromosomes which may differ in different individuals. These fluorescent polymorphisms (see p. 167) are inherited in a simple Mendelian manner and can therefore be used as markers to study the transmission of a particular chromosome from one generation to another.

Finally a recent finding has been that certain viruses may induce aberrations on specific chromosomes *in vitro* (e.g. adenovirus type 12 produces aberrations specifically on chromosome 17) and this technique is now being exploited in chromosome identification (Vause & McDougall, 1973).

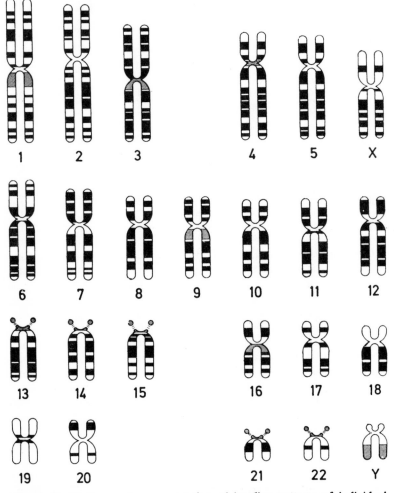

Figure 18. Diagrammatic representation of banding patterns of individual chromosomes as revealed by fluorescent and Giemsa staining (*see* Paris Conference, 1971).

AUTOSOMAL ABNORMALITIES

Within three years of Tjio and Levan's publications there appeared the first of many papers which showed clearly that certain diseases in man are associated with specific chromosome abnormalities.

Chromosome abnormalites can be divided into those which involve the autosomes and those which involve the sex chromosomes. We will first discuss chromosome abnormalities involving the autosomes. These can be subdivided into numerical and structural abnormalities. Numerical abnormalities involve the loss or gain of one or two chromosomes (*aneuploidy*) or even sometimes the gain of a whole chromosome set. The latter condition is referred to as *polyploidy* and is well known to horticulturalists for polyploid varieties of many plants have been recognized for some years. Polyploid cells contain multiples of the haploid (N) number of chromosomes (i.e. $3N$, $4N$, and so on). In man aneuploid and polyploid cells have been found in tissues from some abortuses and stillbirths, in leucocytes from patients with acute leukaemia, and in cancer cells. In cancer cells all manner of numerical and structural chromosome abnormalities occur. Survival after birth with triploid cells in every tissue of the body is extremely rare. Only a few triploid live births have been described and all have died shortly after birth.

Recent studies have shown that variations in the number and structure of chromosomes can be found in *pre*-malignant tissues taken from the cervix. Premalignant tissues are tissues in which there are certain microscopic changes which suggest to the pathologist that the tissue is beginning to undergo malignant transformation but true carcinomatous change has not yet occurred. It is still too early to assess the true significance of these findings but perhaps the causative agent evokes alterations in the chromosomes which are then responsible for all the subsequent pathological changes we associate with malignancy.

Just as polyploidy appears to be lethal in man so does *monosomy* or the loss of an autosome, for no case has been confirmed of an individual with 45 chromosomes due to a deficiency of a whole autosome. Presumably even the very small autosomes carry so many important genes that the loss of such a chromosome is lethal. On the other hand *trisomy*, or the addition of an extra autosome has been described in several disorders in man. In fact the first report of a specific chromosome abnormality associated with a particular disorder was made by Lejeune and his colleagues in Paris in 1959. They showed that patients with Down's syndrome (mongolism) usually have 47 chromosomes; the extra chromosome being a number 21 (fig. 19). Children with Down's syndrome have a characteristic appearance with almond-shaped eyes and a rather roundish head. They are mentally retarded and frequently die young. They have an increased susceptibility to infection, often have congenital heart disease, and an increased frequency of acute leukaemia. They are usually delightful children, easy to manage, and, for some reason, love music. Presumably all these manifestations are a result either directly or indirectly of the genes on the extra chromosome. Recent data suggest that over half of conceptions with trisomy-21 fail to survive to term (Creasy and Crolla, 1974) which indicates that the extra autosome also interferes with intrauterine development.

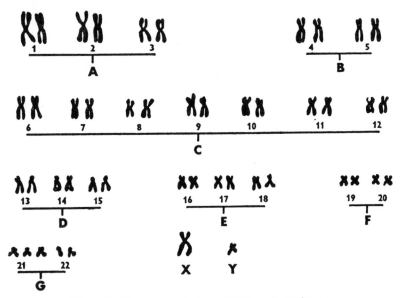

Figure 19. Karyotype of a boy with Down's syndrome.

Other clinical *syndromes* have been described in which there is an extra autosome, a syndrome being a term used in medicine to describe a complex of signs and symptoms which occur together in any particular disorder. In one (Patau's syndrome) there is an extra chromosome 13 and in the other (Edward's syndrome) there is an extra chromosome 18. Both these conditions are comparatively rare; affected babies usually have multiple abnormalities and rarely survive infancy.

Trisomy has been recognized for many years in Jimson weed, maize, tomato, and the fruit fly, and an explanation for the phenomenon was put forward by Bridges in 1916. As we have seen already, the two members of a pair of homologous chromosomes segregate during meiosis, resulting in a haploid set of chromosomes in each gamete. Fortunately accidents rarely occur during this process but occasionally two homologous chromosomes fail to separate (disjoin) and migrate together into the same gamete. This is called *non-disjunction*. Clearly if a gamete containing two chromosomes 21 unites with a normal gamete containing a single chromosome 21 the result will be a zygote which is trisomic for this chromosome. Non-disjunction may occur not only during meiosis in gamete formation but also in the early mitotic divisions of the developing zygote though the former is probably more frequent. In the latter case the corresponding monosomic cells with only one chromosome 21 probably die.

A pair of male twins has been described in which blood group and other studies indicated that they were identical, yet one of them had Down's syndrome. Identical twins arise by the fertilization of a single egg by a single sperm but at an early stage in development the egg divides to form two separate embryos instead of one. Identical twins should therefore have identical genotypes. An explanation for one of a pair of identical twins having Down's syndrome is that possibly non-disjunction occurred at an early cleavage division in one of the embryos.

Occasionally females with Down's syndrome have had children. On average half their children have been normal and half have had Down's syndrome. The reason is that the ova produced by a female with 21-trisomy will be of two types: on the average half the ova will have two chromosomes 21 (secondary non-disjunction) and half will be normal and have only one chromosome 21. The cause of non-disjunction and why certain women have children with Down's syndrome while others do not, is probably the result of an ageing effect on the ova. It has been known for many years that the frequency of Down's syndrome is closely related to the age of the mother: for women who are less than 25 years old the risk of having a child with Down's syndrome is only about 1 in 2000 whereas for some women over 40 years old the chances rise to as high as 1 in 50. A maternal age effect has also been demonstrated in the 13- and 18-trisomies.

In humans, developing ova reach the prophase stage of meiosis I in the fetus and remain at this stage for many years until at ovulation they are shed into the Fallopian tube. Some of the ova will remain at this stage for 40 or 45 years before being shed, and as a consequence it does not seem unreasonable to suppose that ageing might affect them and predispose to non-disjunction. The incidence of Down's syndrome appears to be unrelated to the age of the father. This might be because there is a very rapid turnover of developing spermatozoa throughout reproductive life and thus little time for any ageing process to have an effect. Another factor to be considered is that occasionally more than one child with 21-trisomy may occur in the same sibship which suggests, at least in these cases, that the phenomenon of non-disjunction may be under genetic control. Other factors which have also been implicated as causes of non-disjunction include radiation (e.g. Alberman *et al.*, 1972) and delayed fertilization. In animals it has been shown that aneuploid embryos can result from lengthening the interval between copulation and fertilization, and it has been suggested that this might explain the relationship between, for example, Down's syndrome and maternal age since with increasing age intercourse is likely to be less frequent and delayed fertilization therefore more likely.

Turning now to structural abnormalities of the autosomes, those which have been most clearly defined in man are *translocations* in which there is an exchange of segments between non-homologous chromosomes, and *deletions* in which a segment of a chromosome has been lost. Though the majority of children with Down's syndrome have 47 chromosomes being trisomic for chromosome 21, a few (about 3 per cent) have the normal number of 46 chromosomes. If the chromosomes of one of these children are carefully studied it is found that though the actual number of chromosomes is normal the chromosomes themselves are not normal. The usual finding is that a chromosome in the D (13–15) group is ' missing ' but there is an additional chromosome in the C (6–12) group, and in the mother one of the chromosomes 21 is missing as well. The explanation is that there has been an exchange of chromosome material between a D group chromosome (14 or 15) and chromosome 21 (fig. 20). A large part of the long arm of chromosome 21 is exchanged with a part of the short arm of a D group chromosome. The ' fragment ' formed by the fusion of the short arms of the two chromosomes is lost.

The translocation chromosome, composed of the long arms of a D group and a 21 chromosome, resembles a C group chromosome and this explains why there is an extra chromosome in the C group in both carriers and affected children. A carrier of such a D/G translocation (who has only 45 chromosomes) produces four types of gametes (fig. 20). A gamete may contain a normal D chromosome and a normal chromosome 21 in which case the resulting offspring will be normal. Or a gamete may contain a translocation chromosome (D/G) in which case the resulting offspring will have only 45 chromosomes and will be a carrier like the parent. Or a gamete may contain the translocation and a normal chromosome 21 in which case the offspring will have 46 chromosomes but in effect will be trisomic for chromosome 21 and will therefore have Down's syndrome. Finally a gamete may contain a D chromosome but no chromosome 21; this would produce a zygote monosomic for chromosome 21 which is lethal and would presumably result in an abortion.

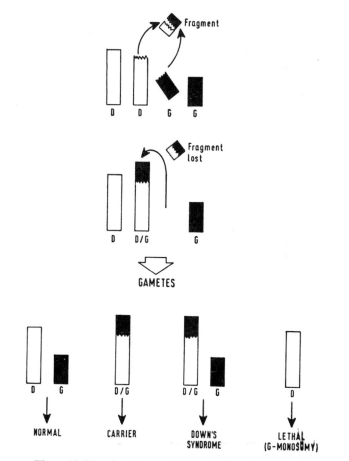

Figure 20. Translocation mechanism in Down's syndrome.

Thus it is important to recognize a carrier of a D/G translocation because there is a theoretical risk of 1 in 3 (but see p. 208) that any particular pregnancy will result in a child with Down's syndrome. Occasionally a parent may carry a translocation which involves a chromosome 21 and a chromosome 22. The genetic risks in these cases are roughly the same as those involving a D/G translocation. However, very rarely a mother may carry a translocation involving both chromosomes 21, in which case all her offspring will have Down's syndrome.

The mother is usually the carrier of the translocation although occasionally the father carries the translocation. However, fathers who carry a D/G translocation rarely have affected offspring. The reason why this should be so is obscure. Genetic counselling in Down's syndrome will be discussed in more detail in chapter 11. It should be realized, however, that in more than half the cases of translocation Down's syndrome, the chromosome abnormality has arisen *de novo,* neither parent carries the chromosome abnormality and the risks of recurrence in subsequent children are small.

Though monosomy of an autosome is apparently lethal, *partial-monosomy* has been recognized in several patients with various congenital abnormalities. In partial monosomy, as the name implies, only a part of an autosome is deficient. This is often referred to as a *deletion.* Deletions of several of the autosomes have been described, some being associated with specific clinical syndromes (table VIII).

In 1963 Lejeune and his colleagues in Paris described a mentally retarded infant with various congenital abnormalities and a characteristic cry which closely resembled the mewing of a cat. For this reason this disorder has since been referred to as the ' cri du chat ' syndrome. This syndrome is associated with a deletion of the short arm of chromosome 5.

An interesting finding has been the recognition of ring chromosomes usually in infants with multiple congenital abnormalities. A ring chromosome indicates that there have been deletions at both ends of a chromosome and that the deleted ends, which are more ' sticky ' have then adhered to each other to form a ring. Ring formation with assumed deletions has been described for several of the autosomes and the X chromosome. At this point mention might also be made of *partial-trisomy* which differs from trisomy proper in that the extra chromosome is partially deleted. One would therefore expect that an individual with an extra, but deleted chromosome 13 would be less severely affected and have only some of the stigmata of the full 13-trisomy syndrome. In fact there have been

Table VIII. *Autosomal abnormalities associated with recognized clinical syndromes*

Chromosome abnormality	Syndrome	Clinical features
trisomy-21 translocation 14 or 15/21 translocation 22/21 translocation 21/21	Down's	characteristic facies mental retardation hypotonia congenital heart disease Simian palmar crease
trisomy-8	——	moderate mental retardation concomitant strabismus clinodactyly other skeletal defects
trisomy-9	——	abnormal facies skeletal abnormalities hypoplastic genitalia congenital heart disease
trisomy-13	Patau's	motor and mental retardation microcephaly microphthalmia cleft palate/hare lip polydactyly congenital heart disease
trisomy-18	Edwards'	motor and mental retardation flexion deformities of fingers micrognathia ' rocker-bottom ' feet congenital heart disease
trisomy-22	——	mental and motor retardation microcephaly abnormal facies and ears
trisomy-4p	——	abnormal facies digital anomalies foot deformities
trisomy-9p	——	abnormal facies large, low-set ears mental retardation incurved and short V digit
4p –	——	mental retardation abnormal facies cleft palate coloboma epilepsy hypospadias scalp defects
5p –	Cri du chat	mental retardation microcephaly hypertelorism characteristic cry

Table VIII. *Autosomal abnormalities associated with recognized clinical syndromes—continued*

Chromosome abnormality	Syndrome	Clinical features
13q− 13r	——	mental and motor retardation abnormal facies microcephaly abnormal thumbs abnormal ears
18q−	De Grouchy's	mental retardation ' carp-mouth ' abnormal ears tapering fingers
18p−	De Grouchy's	mental retardation ocular abnormalities abnormal ears dental decay CNS abnormalities
18r	——	combination of 18p− and 18q− features
21q− (G deletion syndrome I)	' anti-mongolism '	antimongoloid slant of eyes hypertonia micrognathia growth retardation skeletal malformations
22q− (G deletion syndrome II)	——	epicanthic folds hypotonia syndactyly retarded development

several reports of infants with various congenital abnormalities which could be attributed to partial trisomy.

There is a shorthand notation for chromosome abnormalities. Some of the abbreviations now used by cytogeneticists include: *p* and *q* for the short and long arms of chromosomes respectively, *t* for a translocation, *inv* for an inversion, *i* for an isochromosome and *r* for a ring chromosome. The + or − signs are placed *before* the appropriate symbol where they mean additional or missing whole chromosomes, but *after* a symbol where an increase or decrease in length is meant. For example, a male with Down's syndrome due to an additional chromosome 21 is represented as 47, XY, +21 whereas a male with 46 chromosomes and a deletion of the short arm of chromosome 5 is represented as 46, XY, 5p−. A woman with 45 chromosomes and a balanced translocation involving the long arms of chromosomes 15 and 21 is represented as 45, XX, −15, −21, +t (15q 21q).

In 1960 investigators in Philadelphia were the first to describe an abnormal chromosome in blood cultures from patients with a particular type of leukaemia. This abnormal chromosome was later referred to as the *Philadelphia* or *Ph*[1] *chromosome*. It is an acquired chromosome abnormality and is not present at birth. The Ph^1 chromosome is found only in one particular type of leukaemia, namely chronic granulocytic leukaemia. It occurs in blood or bone marrow cells but is not found in skin cells or cells from other tissues which in patients with this disease have a perfectly normal chromosome complement. The Ph^1 is a minute chromosome which is now known to be chromosome 22 with a deleted long arm which has been translocated to the long arm of chromosome 9, i.e. t(22q−; 9q+), or possibly to another autosome.

At first it was thought that the abnormal chromosome might be the cause of leukaemia but this now seems doubtful. Though it has not been established in man, leukaemia can be induced by a virus in mouse and a very potent leukaemia virus has been isolated which produces the disease in 80 to 100 per cent of animals within a few weeks after inoculation. It is therefore possible to study individual mice in which it is known with reasonable certainty that they will eventually develop the disease. Studies of these mice have shown that abnormal chromosomes (the Ph^1 chromosome is not found in mouse leukaemia but other chromosome abnormalities occur) are absent from the blood-forming tissues in the pre-leukaemic and very early stages and appear only when the disease is relatively advanced. It is therefore tempting to think that possibly the Ph^1 chromosome in man is the result rather than the cause of leukaemia. However, the situations in mouse and man may be different. Recent reports suggest for instance that Ph^1 may occasionally be present in man sometime *before* the development of overt leukaemia (i.e. pre-leukaemia).

In acute leukaemia some cells are polyploid while others are aneuploid and structural chromosome abnormalities are often present as well. Similar structural and numerical abnormalities of the chromosomes have been found in the leucocytes of patients who have had deep X-ray therapy for one reason or another. These abnormalities may persist and sometimes can be recognized several years after X-ray therapy. These findings and the fact that in patients who have had deep X-ray therapy there is a small, but nevertheless significantly increased risk of developing leukaemia, suggest that the leukaemia in these patients might be related in some way to the persistence of abnormal chromosomes in the blood. In some severe haematological conditions trisomy–8, and less commonly trisomy–9 or trisomy-10, has been observed in bone marrow cells in some cases.

Incidentally, some investigators have reported finding abnormal chromosomes in the blood of patients after an attack of measles thus implying that the measles virus causes chromosomal damage. Even if cells with abnormal chromosome complements do occur in the blood of patients suffering from measles it is quite probable that these cells would be eliminated by the body without causing any harm.

SEX CHROMOSOME ABNORMALITIES

In 1959 sex chromosome aneuploidy in man was demonstrated for the first time by Jacobs and Strong working in Edinburgh and Ford and his colleagues at Harwell. These investigators found that not all males have an XY sex chromosome constitution or that all females have an XX sex chromosome constitution. The exception to the normal male XY sex chromosome constitution was found in Klinefelter's syndrome, a condition in which affected men are sterile, have very small testes, sometimes have gynaecomastia, and are often mentally retarded (fig. 21). They are sterile because their testes fail to produce spermatozoa. Jacobs and Strong found that these patients have an extra X chromosome, that is, they have an XXY sex chromosome constitution. Other investigators have since shown that males with Klinefelter's syndrome may have as many as four X chromosomes as well as a Y chromosome and cases have been described with an XXYY sex chromosome constitution.

The exception to the normal female XX sex chromosome constitution was found in a condition referred to as Turner's syndrome (fig. 22) in which the affected female is sterile, does not menstruate, is short of stature, and often has various congenital abnormalities such as a web of skin on either side of the neck, coarctation of the aorta, and when the arm is extended the forearm tends to be displaced outward away from the body (cubitus valgus). Ford showed that these women had only one sex chromosome; they had an XO sex chromosome constitution. It is interesting to note that the germ cells in the ovary are normal in early XO fetuses but gradually decline in number during development until at birth germ cells are absent. Klinefelter's syndrome is commoner among the sons of older mothers but such a relationship with maternal age has not been demonstrated in Turner's syndrome.

Females with three or even four X chromosomes have been described. They are sometimes mentally retarded though in all other respects they appear to be perfectly normal females. So far all the

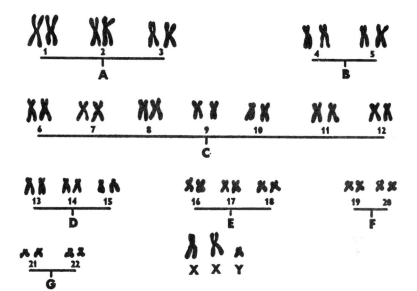

Figure 21. Karyotype of a patient with Klinefelter's syndrome (47, XXY).

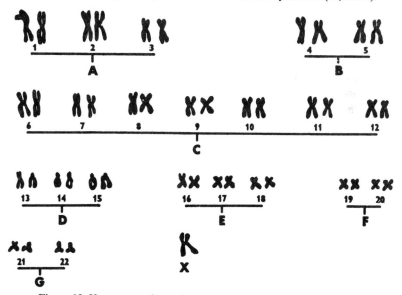

Figure 22. Karyotype of a patient with Turner's syndrome (45, XO).

children of XXX women have been normal in contrast to the off-spring of women with Down's sydrome half of whose children are similarly affected. The reason why females with an XXX sex chromosome constitution (and also males with XYY sex chromosome constitution—see below) have only normal children is not known.

There appears to be a relationship between mental retardation and an increased number of X chromosomes in both phenotypic males and phenotypic females. For example, in Klinefelter's syndrome, all individuals with an XXXY sex chromosome constitution are mentally defective but only about a quarter of those with an XXY pattern are affected in this way. Also patients with an XXXY or XXXXY sex chromosome constitution often have congenital defects not usually seen in XXY cases.

A recent finding has been that men with an XYY sex chromosome constitution occur with increased frequency among the inmates of establishments for the mentally subnormal with criminal propensities. Depending on the method of ascertainment some surveys have found that about 2 to 3 per cent of the inmates of such establishments may be XYY, compared with an incidence of about 1 in 1000 in newborns. Individuals with an XYY sex chromosome constitution tend to be over 6 feet (183 cm.) tall, and to be predisposed to mental subnormality with aggressive antisocial behaviour. The picture is not entirely clear however, because XYY individuals have been found ' by chance ' in the general population and though often tall have not necessarily been delinquent or mentally retarded (Casey et al., 1973). The consequences of an XYY sex chromosome constitution have yet to be fully assessed. However, a recent extensive review suggests that the risk of an XYY male being in custody at some time in life is about 1 in 30, but this is probably influenced very much by the circumstances into which he is born (Hook, 1973).

These sex chromosome abnormalities arise in the same way as in Down's syndrome with 21-trisomy that is, they are the result of non-disjunction having occurred during gametogenesis (fig. 23). Non-disjunction may also occur during early embryogenesis and we shall discuss this later (p. 77). If non-disjunction occurred during oogenesis and the ovum containing no sex chromosomes was fertilized by an X-bearing sperm, the result would be a zygote with an XO sex chromosome constitution. If the ovum were fertilized by a Y-bearing sperm then the result would be a zygote with a YO sex chromosome constitution. This is probably lethal because no individual has ever been found with this sex chromosome pattern. The X chromosome is of maternal origin in about 75 per cent of

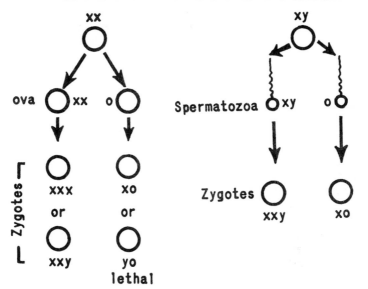

Figure 23. Non-disjunction during oogenesis and spermatogenesis.

individuals with Turner's syndrome, and the two X chromosomes are of maternal origin in about 75 per cent of individuals with Klinefelter's syndrome. Cases with four or more sex chromosomes cannot be explained by a single non-disjunctional event and we have to postulate that two such events have occurred, one during meiosis I and the other during meiosis II. XYY individuals can only result during gametogenesis if non-disjunction occurs at meiosis II, i.e. the Y chromatids fail to separate.

Very rarely double trisomics have been found. Ford has described a child with 21-trisomy and who also had XXY sex chromosome constitution and since then 21-trisomy associated with various other autosomal and gonosomal trisomies have been reported.

Besides tissue culture for chromosome studies, there are four other investigations which may be helpful to the physician in the diagnosis of chromosome abnormalities. These are studies of the sex-chromatin (= X-chromatin) and fluorescent bodies (= Y-chromatin) in buccal smears, examination of 'drumsticks' in polymorphonuclear leucocytes in blood smears, and dermatoglyphics. Gently scraping the inside of the cheek with a tongue depressor is an easy and effective way of obtaining cells for microscopic examination. The scrapings are spread onto a glass microscope slide and then stained. When this is done it is found that in normal women there is a small dark-staining body at the periphery of the nucleus in about half the cells examined. A similar body is not found in normal males. This body is called the X-chromatin body and represents an X chromosome which is inactive and contracted down. Generally speaking, the number of X-chromatin bodies is one less than the number of X chromosomes. The normal female has two X chromosomes and so she has $(2-1) = 1$ X-chromatin body. A patient with XO Turner's syndrome is X-chromatin negative whereas a patient with Klinefelter's syndrome and four X chromosomes (XXXXY) has three X-chromatin bodies. The X-chromatin body is not only found in cells from the lining of the mouth but can be identified in interphase (but not dividing) nuclei from the majority of tissues of the female. The determination of the number of X-chromatin bodies may be very useful in making a diagnosis in patients with abnormalities of sexual development. It has also found use in forensic medicine and sexing unborn babies. As the fetus grows it sheds cells into the amniotic fluid which surrounds it in the uterus. Some of this fluid can be removed during pregnancy and the cells examined for X-chromatin bodies. In this way it is possible to determine, with a high degree of accuracy, the sex of the fetus as early as the third month of pregnancy (p. 215).

The number of Y chromosomes can also be recognized in buccal smears because the Y chromosome fluoresces in the presence of certain dyes such as quinacrine dihydrochloride. By a combination of staining for X-chromatin and Y-chromatin it is possible from the buccal smear to determine a person's sex chromosome constitution.

Another way in which the number of X chromosomes can be determined is by examination of the nuclei of polymorphs in stained peripheral blood smears. About 3 per cent of the polymorphs of females have a small accessory nuclear lobule resembling a drumstick which projects from the main mass of the nuclear lobes. This is not seen in polymorphs from males, or females with an XO sex chromosome constitution. Unfortunately the number of drumsticks is not directly related to the number of X chromosomes when there are more than two: females who are XXX very rarely have two drumsticks.

Dermatoglyphics, or the study of finger prints (dermal ridge patterns), has been used in the identification of criminals for many years, and recently its use has been extended to clinical medicine. Prints obtained from the balls of the fingers and thumbs, the palms, and from the soles of the feet have been studied in a variety of conditions associated with chromosome abnormalities. It has been found that the dermal ridge patterns are often abnormal in Down's syndrome, sometimes abnormal in infants with 13- and 18-trisomy, and occasionally abnormal in women with Turner's syndrome. The abnormal patterns are in no way specific for a particular condition but are sufficiently well defined in certain chromosome abnormalities that they may be very helpful in diagnosis. A small proportion of mothers of children with Down's syndrome also have abnormal dermal ridge patterns.

Let us now consider the function of the sex chromosomes. Apart from one exception, namely the rare condition of hairy ears, no Mendelizing genes are known to be carried on the Y chromosome. That is apart from this one exception, no trait is known which only affects males and is always transmitted from father to son. Yet important genes for normal sexual development must be carried on the Y chromosome because individuals with XO Turner's syndrome are phenotypically female and individuals with as many as four X chromosomes are still phenotypically male if they also have a Y chromosome. On the other hand males with two Y chromosomes are not super-males: as we have seen they tend to be taller and perhaps more prone to delinquency than normal males. The length of the Y chromosome varies from person to person and this variation in size is probably genetically determined.

The Y chromosome is necessary for the development of testes which later produce male hormones with all the attendant masculinizing effects. What happens then, if the testes are removed from a male fetus before the various genital organs have had time to develop? This experiment was actually carried out by Jost some years ago. Jost found that if the testes were removed from male fetal rabbits, they developed into females despite the fact that they were genetically males with an XY sex chromosome constitution. In man there is an interesting condition called the 'testicular feminization' syndrome. Affected persons appear to be perfectly normal females with breasts and female external genitals, but they do not menstruate and are sterile. Chromosome studies of patients with this syndrome have shown that they have an XY sex chromosome constitution and do in fact have testes which are often located in the groin and are sometimes mistaken for a hernia. The reason why these persons appear to be normal females and do not have any outward manifestations of masculinity is believed to be because their tissues are unresponsive to the effects of male hormones synthesized by the testes.

True hermaphroditism is another condition in which there is some ambiguity regarding the sexual status of the individual. All degrees have been described from those who appear to be almost like a normal male to those who appear to be almost like a normal female. There are varying degrees of bisexuality in the genitalia as well as in general physique. When an exploratory operation is carried out on these patients an ovary may be found on one side and a testis on the other. Sometimes there is a mixture of ovarian and testicular tissue (ovo-testes) on both sides or sometimes only on one side, the gonad on the other side being an ovary or a testis. The existence of tissues with different chromosome complements within the same individual is called *mosaicism*. One would expect that true hermaphrodites would be XX/XY mosaics, some of the cells having an XX sex chromosome constitution and others having an XY sex chromosome constitution. In fact some hermaphrodites are XX/XY mosaics but for some reason, which is still not clear, the sex chromosome constitution of many of these patients appears to be XX. However, in most of these cases chromosome studies have been limited to a single tissue, usually peripheral blood, and for this reason mosaicism has not been excluded: other tissues might have an XY sex chromosome pattern. Another possible explanation for XX hermaphrodites is that their paternal X chromosome carries

Table IX. *A classification of various disorders of sexual development*

1. *Seminiferous tubule dysgenesis* (Klinefelter's syndrome)
   XXY, XXXY, etc.
2. *Ovarian dysgenesis* (Turner's syndrome)
   XO
3. *Pseudohermaphrodite*
   (a) male pseudohermaphrodite (XY)
       testicular feminization syndrome
   (b) female pseudohermaphrodite (XX)
       adrenogenital syndrome
4. *True hermaphrodite*
   XX, XX/XY, XX/XO etc.

male determining genes as a result of crossing-over between the X and Y chromosomes during meiosis in spermatogenesis (see Ferguson-Smith, 1965). A useful classification of various abnormalities of sexual development is given in table IX. A good review is to be found in Scott (1971).

The approximate incidences at birth of various chromosome abnormalities is given in table X. The incidence of *major* chromosome abnormalities is approximately 1 in 200 births compared with an incidence of approximately 1 in 400 births with an inborn error

Table X. *Approximate frequencies at birth of various chromosome abnormalities*

	Frequency (per 1000 live births)
1. *Autosomal*	
(a) normal phenotype	
D/G D/D translocations, etc.	2·0
(b) abnormal phenotype	
trisomy–21	1·4
trisomy–13	0·1
trisomy–18	0·1
Others	0·2
2. *Gonosomal*	
XXY	1·3 (in males)
XYY	1·0 („ „)
XXX	1·0 (in females)
XO	0·1 („ „)
Others	0·1

of metabolism and 1 in 50 births with a major congenital abnormality.

HUMAN MOSAICS AND CHIMAERAS

A great variety of mosaics have been described in man. For example, patients with Klinefelter's syndrome have been found with the following sex chromosome constitutions: XX/XXXY, XY/XXY, XY/XXXY, XXXY/XXXXY, or even three different cell lines XY/XXY/XXXY. The patient appears less affected the greater the proportion of cells with a normal male XY sex chromosome complement. Mosaicism has been described not only in patients with Klinefelter's syndrome but also in patients with various other disorders including Turner's syndrome (XO/XX, XO/XXX, XO/XX/XXX, XO/XYY) and Down's syndrome. A child with Down's syndrome who is a mosaic, has two populations of cells in his body. Some cells have a normal chromosome complement with only two chromosomes 21, while others have three chromosomes 21. The greater the proportion of cells with a normal complement of chromosomes, the more likely it is that the child will appear more normal.

There are two ways in which a mosaic might arise. It may be the result of non-disjunction in early embryogenesis with the persistence of more than one cell-line. Thus if a zygote has two X chromosomes and non-disjunction occurs so that one daughter cell receives three X chromosomes (XXX) while the other receives only one X chromosome (XO) this will result in an XO/XXX mosaic. This appears to be the way in which most mosaics arise. However another possible cause of an XX/XY mosaic is double fertilization whereby two genetically different sperms fertilize two egg nuclei and the resulting two diploid nuclei both contribute to the formation of the individual. We now know that this can occur in man from the results of blood group and other studies of the parents of certain patients who are known to be mosaics. Double fertilization must be a rare event.

A distinction has been made between a mosaic and a *chimaera*. In both there is more than one population of cells within the body but whereas in a mosaic they are of the same genetic origin, in a chimaera they are not. A chimaera may be defined as an individual containing two or more genetically distinct cell populations derived from more than one zygote. Chimaeras have been described in man which appear to result from an exchange of cells, via the placenta, between non-identical twins while they are in the uterus. For example 90 per cent of one twin's cells may have an XY sex chromosome constitution and 10 per cent an XX sex chromosome constitution. Most of his red cells may be blood-group A but a few may be blood-group B. On the other hand in his twin sister 90 per cent of her cells may have an XX sex chromosome constitution and 10 per cent may be XY. Most of her red cells may be blood-group B but a few may be blood-group A. Often it is possible to demonstrate that mixing of cells has occurred from the results of other tests, including skin grafting. Normally a skin graft will only ' take ' from an identical twin. However, satisfactory skin grafts can be obtained in non-identical twins if they are chimaeras.

Freemartins in cattle are also the result of substances passing through the placenta from one twin to the other. It has been known for many years that when twin calves of opposite sex are born the female sometimes has incompletely developed genital organs and may even have partially developed male genitals. These calves are freemartins and it was believed that they were the result of hormones passing through the placenta from one calf to the other and since male hormone appears before female hormone the effect was mainly on the female calf. However, recent studies suggest that the cause of freemartins may not be hormonal but may be due to chimaerism of the gonadal tissues.

Chimaeras in plants have been produced by grafting and in this way it is possible to obtain shoots with an epidermis of one species overlying a central core of another species. Chimaeras in animals are very much more difficult to produce experimentally but first Dr Tarkowski at the University of Warsaw, and later others, have successfully produced chimaeras in mice by a unique and fascinating procedure. Fertilized eggs from a pregnant mouse are removed when the eggs are only at the 8-cell stage of their development. Two eggs from two different strains of animals are then squeezed together in a drop of culture medium so that they fuse. After a day or two in culture the united eggs are transplanted into a pregnant mouse where they complete their development. When eggs from a light and a dark strain of mice are fused it is possible to recognize a mosaic pattern of colouring in the resulting chimaera. This technique is proving very useful to those research workers who are interested in studying interactions between different tissues and related problems.

In recent years structural abnormalities of the sex chromosomes have been recognized. These abnormalities include deletions, iso-chromosomes, and ring chromosomes. Of those women attending a hospital for investigation of sterility or because they have never menstruated, chromosome studies have revealed that some have a deleted X chromosome, but this is very rare. We have seen already that most patients with Turner's syndrome have 45 chromosomes and because they have only one X chromosome they are sex-chromatin negative. Despite this, a few cases of Turner's syndrome have been found to be sex-chromatin positive and to have 46 chromosomes. They have two X chromosomes but one is greatly enlarged due to duplication of the long arm and loss of the short arm. This abnormal chromosome is called an *isochromosome* and is believed to result from the centromere having divided transversely instead of longitudinally during cell division. A ring chromosome derived from one of the X chromosomes has also been observed occasionally in women with infertility.

MEIOTIC STUDIES IN HUMAN CHROMOSOMES

So far the discussion has been restricted to studies on somatic chromosomes as seen in mitosis in cultured leucocytes or skin fibro-blasts. With improvements in techniques, cytogeneticists are extending their studies to testicular and even ovarian tissues, as means of studying meiotic chromosomes. Such studies are of particular interest since they may provide information on chromosome re-arrangements which can be recognized by the configuration of paired homologous chromosomes (*bivalents*). Occasionally this may be the best way of recognizing the possible existence of such chromosome abnormalities. For example a chromosome *inversion* whereby a segment of a chromosome is inverted, may not be clear in somatic chromosome preparations but only by the abnormal configuration of chiasmata in meiotic material.

Meiotic studies are perhaps especially valuable in males with a normal somatic karyotype and an unexplained low sperm count.

A significant proportion of such individuals have been found to have a meiotic abnormality as the cause of their sterility (Koulischer and Schoysman, 1974).

EXTRACHROMOSOMAL INHERITANCE

Since the head of the sperm consists almost entirely of nuclear material, the nucleus is the only genetic contribution of the male. However, the egg nucleus is surrounded by abundant cytoplasm. The maternal contribution to her offspring therefore is not only nuclear but also cytoplasmic. This is an important point for there is evidence from animal and plant breeding experiments that though most genes are located on the chromosomes within the nucleus some are free in the cytoplasm. The operation of cytoplasmic factors in the determination of a particular characteristic is suggestive when the offspring always resemble the maternal parent. Male sterility in corn and leaf colour in certain plants have been cited as examples of hereditary characteristics determined by cytoplasmic units. Professor C. D. Darlington coined the term 'plasmagene' for these cytoplasmic units. Plasmagenes, like nuclear genes, are self-replicating and capable of determining certain hereditary characteristics. In man there is no proven case of cytoplasmic inheritance though this has been evoked as a possible explanation for the unusual pedigree patterns observed in spina bifida (p. 131) and in a particular type of hereditary blindness (Leber's optic atrophy). In the latter disease the observation which has suggested the possibility of cytoplasmic inheritance is that affected males rarely, if ever, transmit the disease. The disease is always inherited through women who may or may not be affected.

FURTHER READING

Alberman, E., Polani, P. E., Roberts, J. A. F., et al. (1972). Parental exposure to X-irradiation and Down's syndrome. Ann. hum. Genet. 36, 195–208.

Blank, C. E. (1964). Some aspects of chromosome mosaicism in clinical medicine. Lancet, 2, 903–906.

Casey, M. D., Blank, C. E., McLean, T. M. et al. (1973). Male patients with chromosome abnormality in two state hospitals. J. ment. Def. Res. 16, 215-256.

Chandley, A. C. (1975). Human meiotic studies. In Modern Trends in Human Genetics. Vol. 2. Ed. Emery, A. E. H. pp. 31-82. London: Butterworths.

Creasy, M. R. & Crolla, J. A. (1974). Prenatal mortality of trisomy 21 (Down's syndrome). Lancet 1, 473-474.

Davidson, R. G. (1970). Application of cell culture techniques to human genetics. In Modern Trends in Human Genetics. Vol. 1. Ed. Emery, A. E. H. pp. 143–180. London: Butterworths.

Edwards, R G. and Fowler, R. E. (1970). The genetics of human pre-implantation and development. In Modern Trends in Human Genetics. Vol. 1. Ed. Emery, A. E. H. pp. 181–213. London: Butterworths.

Ferguson-Smith, M. A. (1965). Karyotype-phenotype correlations in gonadal dysgenesis and their bearing on the pathogenesis of malformations. *J. med. Genet.* **2,** 142–155.

Ferguson-Smith, M. A., *et al.* (1973). Assignment by deletion of human red cell acid phosphatase gene locus to the short arm of chromosome 2. *Nature (New Biol.)* **243,** 271–274.

Ford, C. E. (1969). Mosaics and chimaeras. *Brit. med. Bull.* **25**(1) 104–109.

Friedrich, U. & Nielsen, J. (1973). Chromosome studies in 5,049 consecutive newborn children. *Clin. Genet.* **4,** 333–343.

Gartler, S. M., Waxman, S. H. and Giblett, E. (1962). An XX/XY human hermaphrodite resulting from double fertilization. *Proc. natn. Acad. Sci. U.S.A.* **48,** 332–335.

Hook, E. B. (1973). Behavioural implications of the human XYY genotype. *Science* **179,** 139–150.

Insley, J. (1970). Sex chromosome abnormalities in children. *Br. J. hosp. Med.* **4,** 103–110.

Jacobs, P. A. (1969). Structural abnormalities of the sex chromosomes. *Br. med. Bull.* **25**(1), 94–98.

Kjessler, B. (1970). Meiotic studies in the human male. In *Modern Trends in Human Genetics.* Vol. 1. Ed. Emery, A. E. H. pp. 214–240. London: Butterworths.

Koulischer, L. & Schoysman, R. (1974). Chromosomes and human infertility. I. Mitotic and meiotic chromosome studies in 202 consecutive male patients. *Clin. Genet.* **5,** 116–126.

Miller, O. J., Miller, D. A. and Warburton, D. (1973). Application of new staining techniques to the study of human chromosomes. *Prog. med. Genet.* **9,** 1–47.

Pantelakis, S. N., Karaklis, A. G., Alexiou, O., *et al.* (1970). Red cell enzymes in trisomy-21. *Am. J. hum. genet.* **22,** 184–193.

Paris Conference (1971). Standardization in human cytogenetics. *Birth Defects: Orig. Art. Ser.* **8**(7), New York: National Foundation.

Penrose, L. S. and Smith, G. F. (1966). *Down's Anomaly.* London: Churchill.

Polani, P. E. (1969) Abnormal sex chromosomes and mental disorder. *Nature, London.* **223,** 680–686.

Renwick, J. H. (1971). The mapping of human chromosomes. *Ann. Rev. Genet.* **5,** 81–120.

Ruddle, F. H. (1973). Linkage analysis in man by somatic cell genetics. *Nature, Lond.* **242,** 165–169.

Sanger, R. and Race, R. R. (1970). Towards mapping the X chromosome. In *Modern Trends in Human Genetics.* Vol. 1. Ed. Emery, A. E. H., pp. 241–266. London: Butterworths.

Scott, J. S. (1971). Intersex and sex chromosome abnormalities. In *Scientific Basis of Obstetrics and Gynaecology.* Ed. Macdonald, R. R., pp. 275–313. London: Churchill.

Taylor, A. I. (1968). Autosomal trisomy syndromes. *J. med. Genet.* **5,** 227–252.

Valentine, G. H. (1969). *The Chromosome Disorders.* 2nd ed. London: Heinemann.

Vause, K. E. and McDougall, J. K. (1973). Identification of group 'E' chromosome abnormalities in human cells. *J. med. Genet.* **10,** 70–73.

Yamamoto, M. and Ingalls, T. H. (1972). Delayed fertilization and chromosome anomalies in the hamster embryo. *Science* **176,** 518–521.

V

Developmental Genetics

After fertilization, the ovum undergoes repeated mitotic divisions to form the embryo. Specialization of cellular function gradually occurs during this period with aggregation of cells of similar function, resulting in the formation of specialized tissues. Later these various tissues become grouped together to form organs and in this way the fetus develops. The manner in which these various processes occur is the province of embryology. In this chapter we are not concerned so much with the structural changes which occur during development as with the way in which these various processes are under genetic control. This branch of genetics is sometimes referred to as developmental genetics.

FERTILIZATION

In the sea-urchin, meiosis is completed before the sperm enters the egg. This is exceptional, for contrary to what might be expected, in most animals meiosis in the egg is completed only *after* fertilization. In certain intestinal worms fertilization takes place even before meiosis begins, but in most vertebrates meiosis I is completed before the sperm penetrates the egg.

The human female ovary contains many hundreds of eggs or ova. By means of careful dissection and study of ovaries from human female fetuses it has been shown that by the time of birth, the ova have all reached the same stage of division, that is, prophase of meiosis I. The majority of these ova never progress any further but remain at this stage thoughout the reproductive life of the individual. Some ova, however, are destined to be shed into the Fallopian tube, one each month. It is within the Fallopian tube that meiosis I is completed. Only after the sperm has penetrated the egg is meiosis II completed. That meiosis I should be completed only at ovulation and meiosis II only after fertilization implies that these processes are under the control of factors outside the cell, but we have little idea as to the nature of these factors. Human oocytes obtained at the time of ovulation can be cultured in special media and under certain conditions they will complete the various stages of meiosis. This technique opens up a new approach to understanding the factors responsible for controlling meiosis *in vivo*.

After the sperm has penetrated the egg and the process of meiosis has been completed, the two nuclei fuse, thus restoring the diploid number of chromosomes. The fertilized egg, or zygote, now undergoes repeated mitotic divisions to form the embryo. Recently there has been a report that human oocytes have been removed and successfully fertilized *in vitro*. This work may provide a basis for allowing some infertile women to conceive but such experiments also raise serious ethical problems.

THE EARLY STAGES OF DEVELOPMENT

Having described the process of fertilization whereby the sperm nucleus and the egg nucleus unite to produce a diploid zygote, we are now left with a most important question, namely, 'What prevents multiple fertilization?' Nature has, in fact, devised several ways of reducing this possibility. In order to effect fertilization the sperm has to traverse a long and arduous path which includes the cervical canal, uterus, and Fallopian tubes. As a result there is a considerable reduction in the number of sperms which reach the Fallopian tube compared with the number in the upper vagina immediately after copulation. Sperm counts in mice have shown a thousandfold reduction in the number of sperms reaching the Fallopian tube.

Another mechanism which reduces the possibility of multiple fertilization is that the egg itself is invested in a layer of follicle cells (corona radiata) through which the sperm has to penetrate in order to reach the surface of the egg, and the latter itself is surrounded by a thick membrane (zona pellucida) which also has to be penetrated. Once a sperm has penetrated the zona pellucida in many animals a reaction occurs at the egg surface which appears to prevent further penetration of other sperm. Finally, should multiple fertilization occur, in many organisms the consequences (for example, triploidy) are lethal. Most of these observations have been made on animals for little is known of the mechanism of fertilization in man, but it would seem reasonable that these factors may be of importance in preventing multiple fertilizations in man also.

One of the major unsolved problems of biology concerns the way in which cells first come to differ from one another during development. Biologists have tackled this problem by employing such techniques as nuclear transplantation first achieved with any success by Briggs and King in 1952. In recent years Gurdon has shown by a very elegant technique, that if a nucleus, say, from the intestinal epithelium of a tadpole is introduced into an unfertilized frog's egg whose own nucleus has been destroyed by ultraviolet radiation, the egg will develop, in a proportion of cases, into a normal adult frog. The results of such experiments have clearly shown that all genes are retained in all cells and that genes are inactive in those cells in which they are not required. For example, the above experiment shows that the gene for haemoglobin synthesis is retained by an intestinal epithelial cell. Thus the process of cell specialization and differentiation involves the differential activity of genes present in all cells rather than the selective elimination of unwanted genes. Interestingly enough it has often been assumed that in tissue culture, there is *loss* of specialized function (i.e. the reverse of what happens during development) yet recent work has clearly shown that in a number of instances and under certain conditions, specialized function can be demonstrated. For example, the enzyme cystathionine synthetase is normally synthesized by liver but not skin cells yet in tissue culture skin fibroblasts become capable of synthesizing this enzyme.

Another rather interesting finding in work on amphibian eggs has been that the ribosomes used in the early part of embryonic development are those manufactured during oogenesis and no new ribosomes are synthesized until at least the gastrula stage of development. At the time of fertilization the egg is equipped with the genetic information and full protein synthesizing capacity needed for the early stages of development. Subsequent development involves the generation of new genetic information as progressive nuclear differentiation occurs.

Another problem concerns the role of the cytoplasm in cellular differentiation. This problem has been tackled by transplanting the nucleus of a cell carrying out one type of activity into the enucleated cytoplasm of a cell whose nucleus would normally be active in quite another way, e.g. the nucleus from adult brain tissue into the cytoplasm of an unfertilized egg. In all such experiments the transplanted nuclei adopt the functions characteristic of the normal host-cell nucleus. It seems that the egg cytoplasm contains constituents which control gene activity in normal nuclei. DNA polymerase (an enzyme necessary for the incorporation of precursor substances into new DNA) has been implicated as one of the cytoplasmic constituents which are responsible for differential gene activity.

During nuclear and therefore cellular differentiation some genes become inhibited or '*repressed*', as the molecular biologist prefers to call this phenomenon. Thus the genes responsible for synthe-sizing haemoglobin are present in all the cell nuclei of the body but only in the red cells are they active (=*derepressed*). In nerve cells, skin cells, and all other cells the haemoglobin genes are re-pressed. Here we are at the crux of the main problem in develop-mental genetics, that is, the nature of the factors responsible for repression and derepression of gene loci. Before considering the problem at the molecular level we might inquire into some pertinent cytological observations.

CYTOLOGICAL EVIDENCE OF GENETIC CONTROL IN DEVELOPMENT

In chapter I we mentioned that the chromosomes in the salivary glands of certain insects are very much enlarged and have distinc-tive patterns of transverse bands which represent the sites of different genes. During larval development certain bands swell and produce what are called 'puffs', which appear in a characteristic sequence at certain sites on specific chromosomes (fig. 24). Puffs are associ-ated with the synthesis of RNA and evidence suggests that they are

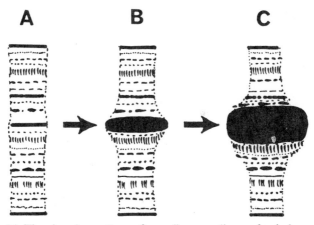

Figure 24. The changing pattern of a puff on a salivary gland chromosome of *Drosophila* during different stages of development.

derepressed genes. Thus in the phenomenon of puffing we have cyto-logical evidence of sequential repression and derepression of genetic loci during the course of development. Ecdysone is a hormone which causes insect larvae to moult and is produced by the prothoracic glands in the larva. The same sequence of puffing which occurs during larval development can be induced in young larvae by injections of ecdysone. In this instance there seems to be an example, at the cytological level, of a chemical substance capable of inducing derepression.

In man there is no comparable cytological evidence of any repression–derepression mechanism apart perhaps from the phenomenon of random inactivation of the X chromosome. This is sometimes referred to as Lyonization of the X chromosome after Dr Mary F. Lyon who was one of the first to propose the hypothesis of X chromosome inactivation. This is perhaps a good point to digress a little and discuss the hypothesis in some detail for it has been a stimulus to much experimental work in human genetics during the last few years. According to this hypothesis there is inactivation of

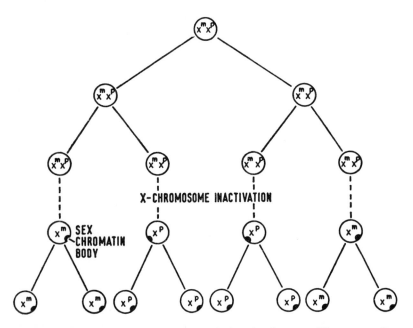

Figure 25. X-chromosome inactivation during development. The maternally and paternally derived X chromosomes are represented as X^m X^p respectively.

all but one of the X chromosomes in each somatic cell (fig. 25). The process of inactivation occurs early in development and in a normal female either of the two X's may become inactivated in different cells of the same individual. (Interestingly, in marsupials the *paternal* X chromosome is consistently inactivated.) Once a particular X chromosome in a particular cell assumes an inactive role, and forms the sex-chromatin body, the same X chromosome becomes inactive in all descendent cells. Since 1961 when the hypothesis was first advanced, there has gradually accumulated much experimental evidence in its favour. It was formulated in order to explain several rather puzzling observations concerning the X chromosome. Cytological studies had shown that in cells of various tissues of female animals one chromosome is darkly stained (heteropyknotic) in interphase nuclei and forms what is called the X-chromatin body. There are a number of valid reasons for considering the X-chromatin body to be one of the X-chromosomes. It is known that the number of X-chromatin bodies per nucleus is one less than the total number of X chromosomes. That is all but one of the X chromosomes is inactivated when an individual has two or more X chromosomes.

The Lyon hypothesis also explains why female mice heterozygous for X-linked genes affecting coat colour have a mosaic phenotype with patches of white and normal coloured fur. In man several X-linked disorders are known in which the heterozygous female has a mosaic phenotype. As an illustration, in ocular albinism the iris and ocular fundus of affected males are completely lacking in pigment but in the heterozygous female careful examination of the ocular fundus reveals a mosaic pattern of pigmentation. Presumably in the unpigmented areas the active X chromosome is the one bearing the gene for ocular albinism. A further example is that of anhidrotic ectodermal dysplasia in which affected males have scanty hair, no teeth, and no sweat glands. In heterozygous females certain patches of skin are smooth and devoid of sweat glands whereas in other areas the skin is perfectly normal.

The Lyon hypothesis has been invoked as a likely explanation for several other observations. For example, until recently there was no really satisfactory explanation for the phenomenon of ' dosage compensation '. That is, the homozygous normal female with two X chromosomes has no more of certain proteins determined by X-linked genes than does the normal male with only one X chromosome (for example anti-haemophilic globulin), and females with several X chromosomes (such as XXX) have no more of these proteins than do normal women with two X chromosomes. Finally, in those X-linked diseases which have been adequately studied, the homozygous affected female is no more severely affected than an affected male who only has the gene in single dose since he has only one X chromosome. Two points worth emphasizing are that the process of inactivation is random with regard to whether the paternally or maternally derived X chromosome is inactivated, and though the process probably occurs in all somatic cells it does not involve the sex cells.

Returning now to the problems of developmental genetics, a study of sex-chromatin in early human embryos has shown that X chromosome inactivation probably occurs no later than the sixteenth day of development when the embryo consists of less than 5000 cells. The relevance of this finding to the present discussion is that here we have cytological evidence in man of gene repression during development. Several observations indicate that almost the whole length of the human X chromosome, and therefore the genes it bears, is inactivated. However, nothing is known regarding the cause of the inactivation or why it occurs at a particular stage in development.

How did such a system evolve? There have been a number of possible explanations but perhaps the most likely is that X-inactivation evolved through X-Y transfer (Lyon, 1974). At first the sex chromosomes were undifferentiated. Later, though similar (homologous) over most of their length, part of the Y became concerned with testicular development while part of the X chromosome became concerned with ovarian development. Later that part of the Y chromosome not involved in testicular development became translocated to the X chromosome thus producing duplication of genes on the long arm of the X which is that part which becomes inactivated in somatic cells in females. It would be expected that the original duplicated genes would have mutated and diverged though some similarity might remain. For example, this would explain the existence of more than one form of certain X-linked disorders, e.g. Duchenne and Becker types of muscular dystrophy, haemophilia A and haemophilia B (Lyon, 1974).

To continue the discussion of cytological observations pertinent to our understanding of developmental processes, consideration should be given to interaction between different cells, and to interaction between cells and their environment. A very important phenomenon of development is that of *embryonic induction* whereby one tissue exerts a determining influence upon the differentiation of another. In vertebrate embryos the best known examples are the ability of the chordamesoderm tissue to induce the overlying ectoderm to form the elements of the central nervous system, and the optic vesicle (an outgrowth from the forebrain) to induce the adjacent ectoderm to form the lens of the eye.

Several ingenious experimental techniques have been developed in order to study these processes. The use of millipore filters makes it possible to deduce something of the physical nature of inducing agents. Thus it has been shown that certain inductive processes are mediated by complex organic molecules which will traverse millipore filters and that actual cytoplasmic contact between the reacting tissues is not necessary. Another technique, which has been used primarily to elucidate the chemical nature of inducing agents, consists of placing extracts of certain adult animal tissues between two pieces of ectoderm which are thereby induced to form various structures. This technique makes it possible to demonstrate that the inducing agent in such a system is probably a complex protein. Another type of experiment consists of incubating embryonic ectoderm in medium in which chordamesoderm has previously been cultured for a few days. Under these conditions the ectoderm is induced to form neural tissue, pigment, and muscle cells. The substance which diffuses out of the chordamesoderm and acts as an inducer on the ectoderm, probably contains RNA and it now seems that the active principle in embryonic induction is a *nucleo-protein*. The results of such experiments suggest that induction is due to a gene product of one cell diffusing out of that cell and then inducing changes in adjacent cells.

Gene activity during growth and development is also influenced by hormones. We have already mentioned the part played by ecdysone during larval development in insects. In the mouse we have an example of a mutant gene whose action is specifically limited to a single cell type which produces a hormone necessary for normal growth and development. The mutant gene, known as *dwarf*, is a recessive which in the homozygous state produces growth retardation. Careful study of these animals reveals that their pituitary glands are considerably smaller than normal. Histology of the pituitary glands of *dwarf* mice shows that the anterior lobe contains almost exclusively small cells with dark-staining nuclei. There is a complete absence of large eosinophilic cells which are a prominent feature of the anterior lobe of normal pituitary glands. Since the eosinophilic cells produce growth hormone their absence accounts for dwarfism in the affected homozygotes. Implantation of normal pituitary cells promotes the growth of *dwarf* mice so that eventually they attain a normal size. Thus in this example we see how a mutant gene specifically affects one particular type of cell and since this cell produces growth hormone the mutant gene has a profound effect on growth and development in general. Still another example from mouse genetics shows that this is not the only way in which growth retardation may be caused. A mutant, known as *pygmy*, also prevents normal growth but in this case implantation of normal pituitary cells has no effect. However pituitary cells from pygmy mice are effective in restoring normal growth in *dwarf* mice. These observations indicate that the pygmy mutant produces sufficient growth hormone but that its tissues are refractory to its effects. Comparable conditions to *dwarf* and *pygmy* varieties of mice occur in man. Individuals with reduced stature but with normal body proportions and sexual activity are referred to as *sexual ateliotic dwarfs*. This condition may be due either to defective synthesis of growth hormone or to a peripheral unresponsiveness to growth hormone as seems to be the case in the Pygmy tribes of Africa. A further example in man is the condition of nephrogenic diabetes insipidus. Normally the renal excretion of water is controlled by an anti-diuretic hormone produced by the posterior lobe of the pituitary. In nephrogenic diabetes insipidus the pituitary gland produces adequate quantities of hormone but the renal tissues are refractory to its effects with the result that there is excessive excretion of water (polyuria).

Many examples are known, both in animal and human genetics, of mutants which so drastically interfere with normal development that death occurs *in utero*. The existence of these ' lethal mutants ' is of significance because it suggests that their normal alleles must be responsible for maintaining normal development. In *Drosophila* several lethal mutants have been studied in detail (lethal giant larvae, *meander* and *translucida*). Each of these mutant genes alters the normal course of events at a specific time in development (the so-called phenocritical period) and the implication is that their normal alleles must be responsible for maintaining normal development at these particular times. One can imagine that during normal embryogenesis the changes which occur are the result of many genes acting in orderly sequence. Should a particular stage in development be affected because a specific gene fails to bring about an important and critical reaction then the whole process thereafter will be disorderly. Many environmental agents are known in animals, and a few in man, which cause congenital abormalities. An agent believed to cause congenital abnormalities is referred to as a *teratogen*. In man such teratogenic agents include radiation during pregnancy, maternal infection with rubella, and treatment during pregnancy with certain drugs such as thalidomide and synthetic progestins (see p. 200). A teratogen usually causes malformations only if exposure occurs at a time when the embryo is sensitive to its effects. Thus thalidomide causes limb deformities and other congenital malformations only when taken during *early* pregnancy. It may be that some of these teratogens act in a way comparable to the mutant genes we have been discussing: they may interfere with processes which are important at certain critical stages in development.

CONTROL OF DEVELOPMENT AT THE MOLECULAR LEVEL

In chapter II we saw how genes are responsible for the synthesis of polypeptides and that this is meditated by messenger-RNA which transfers genetic information from the nucleus to the ribosomes in the cytoplasm where protein synthesis takes place. It was stated that genetic information is stored in the form of a code in the DNA of the chromosomes. In fact the chromosomes are not entirely composed of DNA but also contain a small amount of RNA, calcium and magnesium ions, and certain proteins. These proteins include the *histones* and nonhistone proteins. Recent observations indicate that the histones play a very important part in regulating gene activity. Experiments have shown that in the test tube under appropriate conditions DNA extracted from living tissues is capable of supporting the synthesis of RNA (referred to as ' DNA-dependent RNA synthesis ') and even simple proteins. Now it has been shown that if chromosomal DNA is freed of its histone there is a considerable increase in RNA synthesis as compared with chromosomal material containing histone. From the results of such experiments it now seems clear that in the intact chromosome, histones inhibit DNA-dependent RNA synthesis. That is, histones repress gene action and when the histone is removed the gene is derepressed.

Since the histones would seem to be of such fundamental importance in the regulation of gene activity they are worthy of some further consideration. They were discovered by Miescher who, it will be remembered, was the first to isolate DNA. The histones are basic proteins which contain large proportions of such amino acids as lysine and arginine. Depending on their amino acid composition, four major types have been recognized, but by using various technical refinements at least 50, and possibly as many as 100, different kinds have been found in calf thymus gland which is a rich source of histones. Even if there are 100 different kinds of histone this is still far less than the total number of genes in any one nucleus. For this reason the same histone must be associated with the DNA of several genes, and since the same histones are present in all tissues (except sperm cells) then the same histone must repress different genes in different tissues. There is little doubt that the histones repress gene activity, but it is also possible that other substances in the living cell may have the same effect. Attempts to identify such substances is a field of active investigation at the present moment. Recent work suggests that nonhistone chromosomal proteins may play an important role in gene regulation but exactly how this happens is not known.

The nature of the factors which control tissue or organ growth so that their mass is appropriately related to total body mass is another problem currently being investigated. Recent studies by Bullough and others indicate that active substances (referred to as *chalones*) can be extracted from various tissues which will reversibly inhibit mitosis and this process is potentiated by certain hormones such as adrenaline and glucocorticoids. The chalones are glyco-proteins and are tissue specific but not species specific. Their isolation and characterization is a subject of much interest to developmental biologists. It is possible they may find a place in the treatment of certain types of leukaemia and cancer.

There is increasing evidence that various hormones control the process of development by derepressing gene activity. For instance, it has been known for some time that when animals are treated with certain hormones—cortisone, oestrogens, androgens, or growth hormone—there is an increase in the synthesis of DNA-dependent RNA as well as protein. It seems that hormones function by derepressing certain genes thereby leading to an increase in the synthesis of messenger-RNA and protein.

Let us now consider the relevance of these facts to the genetic control of development. There is a growing belief among present-day biologists that the processes of growth and development are the result of the operation of a network of genetic 'switches'. That is, a particular effector substance (such as a hormone) elicits a

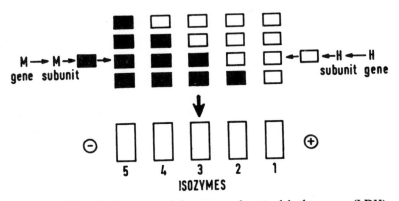

Figure 26. The five isozymes of the enzyme lactate dehydrogenase (LDH). Each isozyme is a tetramer formed from two polypeptide subunits (M and H). The two subunits are synthesized by different genes.

sequence of developmental processes by switching on or off certain genes. Repressed genes may remain repressed or become derepressed depending on their response to the effector substance. In this way certain cells may be rendered susceptible to the action of other effector substances and thereby directed on to new developmental pathways. Other derepressed genes may produce particular enzymes which bring about changes in the metabolism of adjacent cells and tissues.

There are numerous other ways in which it can be imagined that the sequence of events which occur during embryonic development might result from such a system of genetic switches, but much of the detail has yet to be worked out. The observation that many enzymes exist in multiple molecular forms (called *isozymes* or *isoenzymes*) may prove a useful tool for investigating genetic switch mecha-

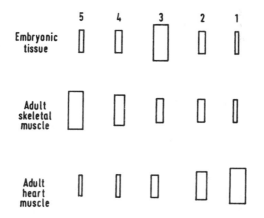

Figure 27. LDH isozyme patterns in embryonic tissues, adult skeletal muscle and adult heart muscle.

nisms during development. The discovery of isozymes was made possible by using the technique of electrophoresis whereby molecules are separated according to their size and electrostatic charge in a gel medium such as starch, agar, or polyacrilamide. The different molecular forms of the enzyme lactate dehydrogenase (LDH), which have been most extensively investigated, are the result of the action of two different genes. These two genes produce two polypeptide subunits, referred to as M and H, which unite together in tetramers to produce five isozymes. The most rapidly migrating isozyme (LDH-1) is composed entirely of H subunits, the most slowly migrating isozyme (LDH-5) of M-subunits and the remaining isozymes

(LDH-2, 3, and 4) of varying proportions of both H and M subunits (fig. 26). In many human embryonic tissues, both the M and H genes appear to be equally active and LDH-3 is the most prominent isozyme. During development, however, in some tissues (e.g. skeletal muscle) the M gene appears to become more active and the proportions of LDH-4 and LDH-5 increase. In other tissues (e.g. heart muscle) the H gene appears to become more active and the proportions of LDH-1 and LDH-2 increase. The patterns seen in adult tissues are present soon after birth (fig. 27).

Since different isozymes predominate in different tissues and at different times in development it would seem that in such a system we have an excellent model for investigating the action of genetic switches during development.

One particularly important application of knowledge of genetic switch mechanisms could be in the treatment of certain genetic diseases. A hint that this might become a real possibility comes from studies on the effects of the drug phenobarbitone. Phenobarbitone is known to induce the synthesis of the enzyme glucuronyl transferase and the drug has been used successfully in the treatment of children with congenital non-haemolytic jaundice (p. 148). Some recent evidence suggests that the disorder can also be prevented if the mother is treated with small doses of phenobarbitone during the later stages of pregnancy.

FURTHER READING

Bell, E. (ed.) (1965). *Molecular and Cellular Aspects of Development*. New York: Harper & Row.

Bonner, J. (1965). *The Molecular Biology of Development*. Oxford: Clarendon.

Bonner, J. and Ts'o, P. O. P. (eds.) (1964). *The Nucleohistones*. San Francisco: Holden-Day.

Briggs, R. and King, T. J. (1960). Nuclear transplantation studies on early gastrulae (*Rana pipiens*). *Devl. Biol.* **2**, 252–270.

Dawson D. M., Goodfriend, T. L. and Kaplan, N. O. (1964). Lactic dehydrogenases: Functions of the two types. *Science, N.Y.* **143**, 929–933.

Ebert, J. D. (1965). *Interacting Systems in Development*. New York: Holt, Rinehart and Winston.

Fischberg, M. and Blackler, A. W. (1961). How cells specialize. *Scient. Am.* **205**(3), 124–140.

Fowler, R. E. and Edwards, R. G. (1973). The genetics of early human development .*Prog. med. Genet.* **9**, 49–112.

Fraser, F. C. (1961). Genetics and congenital malformations. *Prog. med. Genet.* **1**, 38–80.

Gurdon, J. B. (1968). Transplanted nuclei and cell differentiation. *Scient. Am.* **219**(6), 24–35.

Gurdon, J. B. and Woodland, H. R. (1968). The cytoplasmic control of nuclear activity in animal development. *Biol. Rev.* **43**, 233–267.

Grobstein, C. (1959). Differentiation of vertebrae cells. In *The Cell*, vol. 1. Eds. Brachet, J. and Mirsky, A. E., pp. 437–496. New York: Academic Press.

Grüneberg, H. (1967). Sex-linked genes in man and the Lyon hypothesis. *Ann. hum. Genet.* **30,** 239–257.

Hadorn, E. (1961). *Developmental Genetics and Lethal Factors.* New York: Wiley.

Hsia, D. Y. Y. (1968). *Human Developmental Genetics.* Chicago: Year Book Medical Publishers.

Lyon, M. F. (1962). Sex chromatin and gene action in the mammalian X chromosome. *Am. J. hum. Genet.* **14,** 135–148.

Lyon, M. F. (1974). Evolution of X-chromosome inactivation in mammals. *Nature, Lond.* **250,** 651-653.

Maugh, T. H. (1972). Chalones: chemical regulation of cell division. *Science,* **176,** 1407–1408.

McElroy, W. D. and Glass, B. (eds.) (1958). *The Chemical Basis of Development.* Baltimore: Johns Hopkins Press.

Merimee, T. J., Hall, J. D., Rimoin, D. L. and McKusick, V. A. (1969). A metabolic and hormonal basis for classifying ateliotic dwarfs. *Lancet,* **1,** 963–965.

National Cancer Institute Monographs No. 38 (1973). *Chalones: concepts and current researches.* Washington, D.C.: U.S. Government Printing Office.

Saxén, L. and Rapola, J. (1969). *Congenital Defects.* New York: Holt, Rinehart and Winston.

Shaw, C. R. (1965). Electrophoretic variation in enzymes. *Science, N.Y.* **149,** 936–943.

Spratt, N. T. (1965). *Introduction to Cell Differentiation.* London: Chapman and Hall.

Waddington, C. H. (1962). *New Patterns in Genetics and Development.* New York: Columbia University Press.

VI

Inheritance in Families

In man if we wish to investigate the genetics of a particular trait then we usually have to rely mainly on our observations of the manner in which the trait is transmitted from one generation to another, or study the disease among relatives of affected persons. However, most diseases which are inherited in a simple manner are very rare. The common familial diseases usually follow no simple pattern of inheritance.

There are other important reasons for studying inheritance within families apart from helping us to understand the way in which certain diseases are inherited. A thorough knowledge of the manner in which a particular disorder is inherited is essential when giving advice to members of a family regarding the likelihood of their being affected or having affected children. Also the family history often helps in diagnosis. As an example, a child might be brought to the physician because his parents are concerned about the number of times the child has sustained a fracture after seemingly trivial injuries. During the examination the physician asks if anyone else in the family has been affected in this way. If there is a positive family history, that is, if several relatives have been similarly affected, then the physician would probably diagnose osteogenesis imperfecta, a disease known to ' run in families ' as we shall see later. In this example, a knowledge of the family history would suggest the correct diagnosis. In the absence of a positive family history then other diagnoses would have to be considered.

The drawing-up of a family tree or pedigree chart begins with the affected person first found to have the trait, and through whom the family came to the attention of the investigator. This person is referred to as the *propositus,* if a male, and *proposita* if a female. In the pedigree chart the position of the propositus (or proposita) is indicated by an arrow. The next step is to ask whether any brothers or sisters (*sibs*) have been similarly affected, and after careful questioning, the health of all maternal and paternal relatives is carefully recorded and relevant information included on the pedigree chart (fig. 28).

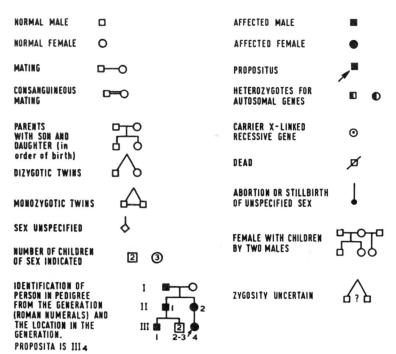

Figure 28. Symbols used in pedigree charts.

A trait which is determined by a gene on an autosome is said to be inherited as an autosomal trait and may be dominant or recessive. A trait which is determined by a gene on one of the sex chromosomes is said to be sex-linked and may also be either dominant or recessive.

AUTOSOMAL DOMINANT INHERITANCE

A dominant trait is one which manifests itself in the heterozygote. That is, a person with an autosomal dominant trait possesses the abnormal (mutant) gene which causes the disorder as well as the normal gene or allele. This is true for *rare* genes but if the mutant gene is common then it is possible that some affected individuals might be homozygous for the mutant gene. However, for rare autosomal dominant genes affected persons are almost always heterozygotes. For the sake of simplicity we will concern ourselves only with rare genes.

In autosomal dominant traits each affected person usually has an affected parent (fig. 29). But this is not always true. Sometimes the disorder may suddenly appear in one generation when no one

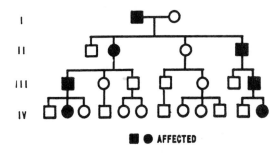

Figure 29. Pedigree pattern of an autosomal dominant trait.

else in earlier generations of the family has been affected. There are several explanations for this. It might be because of illegitimacy, or because one of the parents may in fact have been affected, but so mildly that it was not detected. But, excluding these possibilities, the most likely explanation is that the affected person is equivalent to a 'sport' in horticulture—the sudden unexpected appearance of a new variety. The cause is the same in both instances; they arose as a result of a new *mutation*. A mutation is a change in a gene. As an example, in osteogenesis imperfecta, instead of producing normal bone, the mutant gene produces brittle bones. In many cases of osteogenesis imperfecta there is a history of other members of the family having been affected in previous generations, but occasionally cases arise as a result of a new mutation. The same is true of achondroplasia, a form of dwarfism. In more severe diseases affected individuals only occasionally have children. They may not live long enough to have a family, or may survive but are infertile. In either case the disease ultimately becomes extinct in the family and such diseases are maintained in the population by new mutations occurring in other families.

In a disorder which has little effect on survival it is often possible to trace the disease through many generations. This is true of porphyria variegata (syn: South African porphyria), a metabolic disorder, important manifestations of which are increased sensitivity of the skin to sunlight and the excretion of 'port-wine' coloured urine due to the presence of porphyrins. In South Africa over 8000 cases are known and all these have been traced back to one couple who married in 1688. An even milder condition, inherited as an autosomal dominant trait is brachydactyly (short fingers) which causes no inconvenience to affected individuals. Brachydactyly can often be traced back over many generations. It was the first example in man of a trait which behaved as a Mendelian dominant, as was shown in the early 1900s by Farabee, who was at that time a graduate student at Harvard.

In autosomal dominant traits, if an affected individual marries a normal person, on the *average* half their children will be affected. The reason is that in an affected person each gamete carries either the gene for the trait or the normal gene. All the gametes of the unaffected partner will carry the normal gene. If we represent the dominant (mutant) gene as 'A' and the recessive (normal) gene as 'a' then the various gametic combinations can be represented as:

Affected parent (Aa)
↓
gametes

		A	a
Normal	a	Aa affected	aa normal
parent → gametes			
(aa)	a	Aa affected	aa normal

Since human beings usually have small families with only two or three children, *by chance* an affected person may well have all normal children. On the other hand, again by chance, he may be unlucky and all his children may be affected. Nevertheless on the *average* half the offspring of any affected individual will be affected.

A condition inherited as an autosomal dominant trait affects both males and females.

Autosomal dominant traits tend to be extremely variable in expression. This variability in clinical manifestations is sometimes referred to as *expressivity*. In polydactyly, for example, there may be no more than a small wartlike appendage on the side of the hand but at the other extreme another affected person may have a complete extra finger. In osteogenesis imperfecta some individuals may be so mildly affected that the condition hardly affects their everyday life, but others may be so severely affected that they may become complete invalids with gross skeletal deformities. Most affected individuals lie somewhere between the two extremes. Sometimes a gene may not express itself at all, in which case it is said to be *non-penetrant* and this explains apparent 'skipped' generations in certain pedigrees. Such variations in the expression of a mutant gene are the result of the modifying effects of other genes as well as environmental factors on the expression of the mutant gene.

Some autosomal genes are expressed more frequently in one sex than another. This is called *sex influence*. In the extreme, when only one sex is affected, this is referred to as *sex limitation*. Gout and presenile baldness are examples of sex-influenced autosomal dominant traits, males being predominantly affected in both cases. The influence of sex in these two examples is probably through the effects of male hormones. Gout, for example, is very rare in women before the menopause but the frequency increases in later life. Hippocrates is favoured with having been among the first to note that 'eunuchs neither get gout nor grow bald'. Sex limitation in which *only* one sex is affected would explain pedigrees of testicular feminization syndrome (p. 75). However, since males with this disorder do not reproduce such pedigrees are also compatible with X-linked recessive inheritance (p. 104) which is perhaps more likely since a biochemically similar disorder is known to be X-linked in mouse.

Autosomal Recessive Inheritance

As in the case of autosomal dominant traits, autosomal recessive traits affect both sexes (fig. 30). However, recessive traits are only manifest when the gene is present in double dose, that is, in persons homozygous for that particular mutant gene. Usually heterozygotes are perfectly healthy and all the offspring of an affected person are normal, unless the affected person marries a heterozygote, but be-

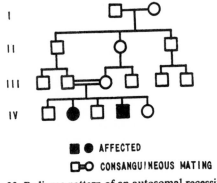

■ ● AFFECTED

□=○ CONSANGUINEOUS MATING

Figure 30. Pedigree pattern of an autosomal recessive trait.

cause of the rarity of most recessive traits this would be very unlikely. Of course, if two affected persons homozygous for the same
gene marry then all their children would be affected, but again such
an event would be very unlikely. In general, both the parents and
the offspring of persons homozygous for a rare recessive gene are
perfectly healthy. The pedigree pattern thus differs considerably
from that found in autosomal dominant traits. It is not possible to
trace the disease through several generations; all the affected individuals in a family are in one *sibship*, that is, they are brothers and
sisters.

About one-quarter of the offspring of two heterozygotes will be
affected. The reason why one-quarter should be affected is because
each parental gamete carries either the gene for the trait or the
normal allele. If we represent the normal gene (which in this case
is dominant) as 'A' and the recessive (mutant) gene as ' a ' then the
various gametic combinations can be represented as:

Normal heterozygous
parent (Aa)
↓
gametes

		A	a
		AA normal	Aa unaffected heterozygote
Normal heterozygous → gametes parent (Aa)	A		
	a	Aa unaffected heterozygote	aa affected

We can see from this that one-quarter of the progeny will be
normal, one-half will be unaffected heterozygotes, and one-quarter
will be affected. As in the case of autosomal dominant traits these
are *average* figures. Two heterozygotes may marry and, if they have
only one child the chances are that it will not be affected. From
theoretical considerations it can be calculated that with regard to
marriages between two heterozygotes, in three-quarters (75 per cent)
of families with only one child that child will be unaffected, in
nine-sixteenths (56 per cent) of families with two children both
children will be unaffected, but in only $\frac{81}{256}$(32 per cent) of families
with four children will all four children be unaffected (table XI).

Therefore by chance some marriages between heterozygotes will result in all normal children and this has to be taken into account in calculating the proportion of affected individuals. There are mathematical devices for doing this. If such precautions are not taken the proportion of affected individuals will not equal the expected value of one-quarter but will be significantly greater since families with no affected children will not have been included in the calculations.

Table XI. *The proportions of families of various sizes with different numbers of affected children*

Number affected	Number of children in sibship			
	1	2	3	4
0	3/4	9/16	27/64	81/256
1	1/4	6/16	27/64	108/256
2	—	1/16	9/64	54/256
3	—	—	1/64	12/256
4	—	—	—	1/256

With *rare* recessive traits, the parents of affected individuals are often related, the reason being that cousins are more likely to carry the same genes because they received them from a common ancestor. In fact the chance that first cousins will carry the same gene is 1 in 8. The chance that two unrelated persons carry the same gene is much less than 1 in 8 though the exact figure depends on the frequency of the gene in the general population. Fibrocystic disease of the pancreas is the commonest autosomal recessive trait known in man, affecting about 1 in every 2000 births. The various manifestations of this disease can largely be accounted for by increased viscosity of the secretions of mucous glands throughout the body. In fact, another name for this condition is mucoviscidosis. In newborn babies affected with this condition the thickened secretions may cause intestinal obstruction (meconium ileus). During infancy and childhood there is interference with the digestive processes resulting in malnutrition and weight loss. The lungs are also affected and pneumonia is a common cause of death. Only about 2 to 3 per cent of adult males with fibrocystic disease are fertile, the cause of their sterility being due to abnormalities of the epididymis, vas deferens, and seminal vesicles resulting in mechanical obstruction to the transport of sperm from the testes to the urethra (Taussig *et al.*, 1972). The majority of affected females have apparently normal fertility.

About 1 person in every 22 carries the gene for fibrocystic disease. The chances that two persons, both heterozygous for this disease, will meet and marry are thus considerably greater than for a much rarer condition such as alkaptonuria, the gene for which is carried by only 1 person in every 500 in the general population (p. 164). Generally speaking, the rarer a recessive disease the greater the frequency of consanguinity among the parents of affected individuals. It was by this reasoning that Bateson suggested in 1902 that alkaptonuria in man was a rare recessive trait (p. 10). Other examples of autosomal recessive traits include many inborn errors of metabolism (p. 27), certain types of deaf-mutism and blindness. At present the frequency of first cousin marriages in the general population of the U.K. is about 0·5 per cent, that is, about 1 in every 200 marriages is between first cousins. In fibrocystic disease of the pancreas the frequency of consanguinity is little greater than in the general population, in albinism roughly 1 in 20 are first cousins, and in alkaptonuria, which is an exceedingly rare condition, a quarter or more of the parents are first cousins.

Because of the nature of their affliction deaf-mutes are often thrown into the company of others who are similarly afflicted and marriages between two affected persons are not uncommon. As we said earlier, one would expect that if two persons homozygous for a recessive condition were to marry and have children, all their children would be affected, but this is not so in every case. A few families have been described in which all the children born to deaf-mute parents have been perfectly normal. This has also been found in some families with certain other recessive conditions such as albinism. The explanation must be that the parents were not homozygous for the *same* gene and that different genes may cause very similar diseases. It is not unreasonable to suppose that mutations at different sites in the DNA molecule might by chance produce similar amino-acid substitutions which result in similar phenotypes. It is also possible that two diseases only appear to be the same condition. In one family in which both parents were albinos and whose children were normal, careful examination of the father revealed that he had a different type of albinism from his wife. The depigmentation in the father was more localized and less marked.

INTERMEDIATE INHERITANCE

In some genetic traits the heterozygote differs from individuals homozygous for the normal gene and also from individuals homozygous for the mutant gene. Intermediate inheritance is a term sometimes applied to this type of inheritance and the gene which is partially expressed in the heterozygote is said to be *incompletely dominant*. For example, the often fatal disease of sickle-cell anaemia results when a person is homozygous for the gene for haemoglobin S. Individuals heterozygous for this gene appear normal and do not usually suffer from any ill effects unless they are exposed to a low concentration of atmospheric oxygen. Air travel at high altitudes in unpressurized aircraft has been known to cause severe damage to the spleen in these persons. Generally speaking, however, heterozygotes are usually perfectly healthy but if a specimen of their blood is withdrawn and exposed to a low concentration of oxygen in a test tube then the red cells lose their normal spherical shape and appear sickle-shaped. Such persons are said to have sickle-cell *trait* rather than sickle-cell anaemia.

If a pedigree of a family with sickle-cell anaemia is drawn up to show only those affected with the anaemia then it appears to be inherited as a recessive. But if those with the trait are also represented then the disease appears to be inherited as a dominant. This demonstrates the arbitrary nature of the concepts of dominance and recessiveness which refer only to phenotypic manifestations and not to the primary gene action. Dominance or recessiveness are not qualities of the gene itself.

Codominance is another term sometimes used for two traits which are both expressed in the heterozygote. In persons with blood group AB it is possible to demonstrate both A and B blood-group substances. The A and B blood groups are therefore codominant. By analysis of the haemoglobin from red cells of persons with sickle-cell trait, it is possible to demonstrate the presence of both haemoglobin A and haemoglobin S. One day we may be able to detect, by appropriate biochemical tests, the presence of the mutant gene in all heterozygotes. This will be dealt with later in Chapter XI.

Sex-linked Inheritance

Sex-linked inheritance refers to the pedigree pattern of genes carried on either of the sex chromosomes. Genes carried on the X chromosome are referred to as being X-linked. Genes carried on the Y chromosome are referred to as being Y-linked. Another term which is occasionally used is that of *partial sex-linkage*. This refers to genes carried on what are believed to be homologous portions of the X and Y chromosomes and it has been suggested that during meiosis pairing occurs between the homologous portions of the sex chromosomes and as a result of crossing-over a gene might be transferred from the X to the Y chromosome or vice versa. There is some evidence for partial sex-linkage in certain animals, but the evidence for partial sex-linkage in man is far less compelling. Partial sex-linkage has been proposed as a possible explanation for certain diseases which appear to be X-linked in some families, Y-linked in others and show a 'confused' pattern of inheritance in yet other families presumably because of crossing-over between the two sex chromosomes. Diseases which have been thought to exhibit partial sex-linkage include total colour blindness (a complete inability to recognize colours, only shades of light and dark being distinguishable) and certain rare skin disorders. But it is extremely difficult in human pedigree data to distinguish between partial sex-linkage and autosomal inheritance. In man partial sex-linkage is an interesting possibility but as yet there is no conclusive evidence for it.

An X-linked recessive trait is one determined by a gene carried on the X chromosome and manifest in the female only when the gene is in double dose, that is in the homozygous state. In the male, a mutant gene carried on the single X chromosome is always manifest because there is no normal gene to counteract the effects of the mutant gene as there is in the heterozygous female. The male with a mutant gene on his single X chromosome is said to be *hemizygous* for that gene since neither of the terms heterozygous nor homozygous are appropriate in this situation. Heterozygous females are usually unaffected. Diseases inherited in this way are therefore transmitted by affected males and by healthy female carriers (figs. 31 and 32).

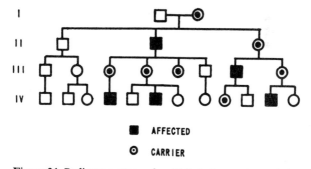

■ AFFECTED

◉ CARRIER

Figure 31. Pedigree pattern of an X-linked recessive trait in which affected males reproduce.

A good example of an X-linked recessive trait is haemophilia. In the past, death of haemophiliacs often occurred in childhood as a result of a minor trauma but with blood transfusion and improve-

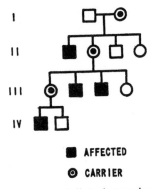

■ AFFECTED

◉ CARRIER

Figure 32. Pedigree pattern of an X-linked recessive trait in which affected males do not reproduce.

ments in surgical techniques affected males can now live an almost normal existence provided they are careful. In the case of an affected male who marries a normal female, if we represent the haemophilia gene as X^h, the various gametic combinations can be represented as shown below:

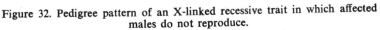

Affected male (X^hY)
↓
gametes

		X^h	Y
Normal female → gametes (XX)	X	XX^h carrier daughter	XY normal son
	X	XX^h carrier daughter	XY normal son

From this we see that since a male transmits an X chromosome to each of his daughters and a Y chromosome to each of his sons, then all the daughters of an affected male will be carriers but none of his sons will be affected. An X-linked trait is never transmitted from a father to his son. In the case of a carrier female marrying a normal male, the various gametic combinations can be represented as:

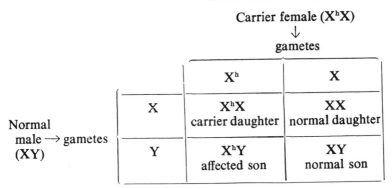

Carrier female (X^{h}X)

From this we see that, with regard to the offspring of a mother who is a carrier, half her sons will be affected and half her daughters will be carriers like their mother.

The mode of inheritance whereby only males are affected by a disease which is transmitted by normal females (this has been called Nasse's law) was appreciated by the Jews nearly 2000 years ago. They excused from circumcision the sons of all the sisters of a mother who had a son with the ' bleeding disease '. The sons of the father's sibs were not excused. Queen Victoria was a carrier of haemophilia and her carrier daughters, who were perfectly healthy, introduced the gene into the Russian and Spanish Royal families. Fortunately for the British Royal family. Queen Victoria's son, Edward VII, did not inherit the gene, and so could not transmit it to his descendants.

Other examples of X-linked recessive traits include partial colour blindness (an inability to distinguish between shades of red and green), testicular feminization syndrome (p. 75), deficiency of the enzyme glucose-6-phosphate dehydrogenase (G6PD), and one form of muscular dystrophy (so-called Duchenne muscular dystrophy). Many other X-linked recessive conditions are known in man but the majority are much rarer than the examples given here. About 8 per cent of males are colour blind but only about 1 woman in 150 is affected because, with rare exceptions, a woman can only be colour blind if she is homozygous for the gene. The enzyme glucose-6-phosphate dehydrogenase is important in cell metabolism. The absence of this enzyme from the red cells renders a person liable to attacks of haemolysis whereby the red cells are destroyed and a severe, even fatal, anaemia results. Males are predominantly affected. Heterozygous females are usually healthy but often have reduced amounts of enzyme in their red cells. G6PD deficiency is particularly common in Negroes and people from Mediterranean countries but is rare elsewhere in the world. These racial differences are of great significance and will be discussed later (p. 167). The fourth example of an X-linked recessive trait is that of Duchenne muscular dystrophy, so named after Guillaume Benjamin Amand Duchenne, who first described the condition in 1868.

Duchenne muscular dystrophy is the commonest form of that group of hereditary diseases which primarily affect the muscles and are referred to collectively as the muscular dystrophies. It is a severe disease coming on gradually during early childhood. One of the first signs is a tendency to waddle from side to side when walking. In the early years affected boys have difficulty in climbing stairs unaided and complain of falling over easily. By about the age of 10 they can no longer walk and have to use a wheel chair. The muscle weakness gradually progresses and ultimately they become confined to bed and usually die before reaching the age of 20. This disease illustrates another point concerning X-linked inheritance. Since affected boys do not survive, the disease is transmitted entirely by healthy female carriers (see fig. 32). Sometimes there is a history of a maternal uncle or other maternal relative having been similarly afflicted, but often the case is the only one in the family. About a third of these ' sporadic ' cases are the result of new mutations.

The pattern of inheritance of an autosomal dominant trait is a vertical one, with affected persons in successive generations, and that of an autosomal recessive trait is horizontal, with affected persons all in the same generation. The pedigree pattern of an X-linked recessive trait in which affected males do not reproduce tends to be oblique because the trait is transmitted to the sons of normal carrier sisters of affected males.

Very rarely a woman may exhibit an X-linked recessive trait. There are several explanations as to how this might happen. First, she might have an XO (Turner's syndrome) or XY (testicular feminization syndrome) sex chromosome constitution; indeed, cases have been described of women with haemophilia or Duchenne muscular dystrophy who had only a single X chromosome. Second, she might be a homozygote because her mother was a carrier and her father was affected, or because her father was affected and her mother was normal but a mutation occurred on the X chromosome she transmitted to her daughter, or her mother was a carrier and her father was normal but a mutation occurred on the X chromosome he transmitted to his daughter. The final possibility is that she might be a 'manifesting heterozygote'. That is she is a heterozygote but because of random inactivation ('Lyonization', see p. 86) by chance in most of her cells the active X chromosome is the one bearing the mutant gene. It is sometimes possible to distinguish between an affected woman who is a homozygote and one who is a manifesting heterozygote. All the sons of a homozygous female will be affected but if a woman has but one normal son she must be a heterozygote. Also homozygous females are as severely affected as hemizygous males but manifesting heterozygotes are usually only slightly affected.

Just as there are dominant and recessive autosomal traits, so there are dominant as well as recessive X-linked traits. An X-linked dominant trait is manifest in the heterozygous female as well as in the male having the mutant gene on his single X chromosome (fig. 33). The pattern of inheritance superficially resembles that of an

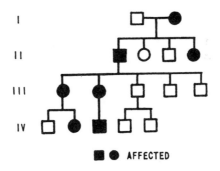

Figure 33. Pedigree pattern of an X-linked dominant trait.

autosomal dominant trait because an affected female transmits the disease to half her sons and to half her daughters but there is an important difference. With an X-linked dominant trait an affected male transmits the disease to *all* his daughters but to *none* of his sons. Therefore in these families there is an excess of affected females. Examples of X-linked dominant traits are vitamin-D-resistant rickets and the Xg blood group. Rickets is due to a deficiency of calcium or vitamin D. But in vitamin-D-resistant rickets, as the name implies, rickets occurs even when there is an adequate intake of vitamin D. Affected persons are refractory to normal doses of vitamin D. In the X-linked dominant form of vitamin-D-resistant rickets both males and females are affected though the females usually have less severe skeletal changes than the males.

With regard to the Xg blood group, persons whose blood reacts with a specific antiserum to Xg blood-group substance are said to be Xg (a +). Those persons who do not react are said to be Xg (a –). Xg (a +) is dominant to Xg (a –) and heterozygous females are therefore always Xg (a +). About 90 per cent of females and 60 per cent of males are Xg (a +).

Holandric or Y-linked inheritance implies that only males are affected and that an affected male transmits the trait to all his sons but to none of his daughters. In the past it has been suggested that such bizarre-sounding conditions as porcupine skin, hairy ears, and webbed toes are Y-linked traits. With the possible exception of hairy ears, the original claims of holandric inheritance in these conditions have not stood up to more careful study.

MULTIPLE ALLELES

So far each of the genetic traits we have considered has involved only two alleles—the normal and the mutant. For example in osteogenesis imperfecta there is the normal gene which leads to normal bone formation and the mutant gene causing brittle bones. Some genes exist in more than two allelic forms, however. Such multiple alleles are the result of a normal gene having mutated to produce various different genes, some of which are dominant and others recessive to the normal gene. In the case of the ABO blood groups there are at least four alleles (A_1, A_2, B and O). An individual may possess any two of these alleles which may be the same or different A_1O, A_2B, OO, and so on). Since alleles are carried on homologous chromosomes a person transmits only one allele for a certain trait to any particular offspring. For example, if a person has the genotype A_1O (phenotypically A_1 since this allele is dominant to O) he will transmit to any particular offspring either the A_1 allele or the O allele but never both or neither (table XII). Certain haemoglobin types constitute an allelic series and one interpretation of the rhesus blood-group system is that it also consists of a series of alleles at one locus.

The preceding remarks concerning the inheritance of multiple alleles relate only to alleles borne on the autosomes. If a series of alleles were carried on the X chromosome then a woman would have two, either of which she might transmit to a particular offspring, whereas a man would only have one allele to transmit. Duchenne muscular dystrophy may represent an allele for normal muscle development, a recessive allele which results in the severe type of X-linked muscular dystrophy and another, but very rare, recessive allele which results in a mild type of X-linked muscular dystrophy (Becker type).

MULTIFACTORIAL INHERITANCE

During the preceding discussions it has been tacitly assumed that each particular inherited trait or disease was the result of the action of a single gene (unifactorial) though occasionally the expression of the gene may be modified by the action of other genes. There are many fairly common conditions, however, in which there is a definite familial tendency, the proportion of affected relatives being greater than in the general population, but the proportion of affected relatives is often of the order of 5 per cent and therefore much less than would be expected for a unifactorial trait. It has sometimes been suggested that the low familial incidence in such conditions might be because the responsible gene was 'incompletely penetrant'.

Table XII. *Possible genotypes, phenotypes, and gametic types formed from the four allelic genes* A_1, A_2, B and O

Genotypes	Phenotypes	Gametes
A_1A_1	A_1	A_1
A_2A_2	A_2	A_2
BB	B	B
OO	O	O
A_1A_2	A_1	A_1 or A_2
A_1B	A_1B	A_1 or B
A_1O	A_1	A_1 or O
A_2B	A_2B	A_2 or B
A_2O	A_2	A_2 or O
BO	B	B or O

This explanation, however, is rather unsatisfactory for several reasons and it is much more likely that such conditions are caused by many genes (polygenic) plus the effects of environment, so-called *multifactorial* inheritance. Normal traits which are inherited in this way include intelligence, stature, skin colour, total dermal ridge count, certain components of ocular refraction and possibly blood pressure. Abnormal traits which may be inherited in this way include certain congenital abnormalities, hypertension, diabetes mellitus, ankylosing spondylitis, rheumatoid arthritis, peptic ulcer and ischaemic heart disease (see chapter VIII). Each of these characteristics is believed to be the result of the action of many genes each of small but additive effect plus the effects of environment (but other explanations are also possible, see Morton *et al.*, 1970). Fisher showed in a classical paper published in 1918, that such a mode of inheritance is really an extension of, and not contrary to Mendelian concepts concerning unifactorial inheritance.

A frequency distribution curve presents in graphic form measurements of a particular characteristic on a number of people in a population. In the case of a trait determined by two genes one of which is dominant to the other, there will be two classes of persons, those manifesting the dominant phenotype and those manifesting the recessive phenotype. The frequency distribution curve is said to be discontinuous and has two humps. If the heterozygote were different from the two homozygotes then the frequency distribution curve would have three humps. However, in multifactorial inheritance there are many genes with no dominance: where the trait can be measured and produces a graded effect the frequency distribution is a smooth, bell-shaped curve—the so-called normal (or Gaussian) distribution. For example in the case of intelligence, at one end of the distribution curve are those persons with limited intelligence and IQ's of less than 60. At the other end of the distribution curve are a few highly intelligent people with an IQ of more than 140, but the majority are somewhere in between—represented by the central portion of the bell-shaped curve. With such normal traits as intelligence there is a tendency for offspring to ' regress toward the norm '. That is, for offspring to have on average values which lie between their parents' and the population averages.

In disease traits, however, although patients can be graded according to the severity of their symptoms, it is not possible to grade them according to their degree of normality. However it is possible in certain diseases to assume that there is some underlying graded attribute which is related to causation. This is referred to as the individual's *liability*, which includes not only his genetic predisposition but also the environmental circumstances which render him more or less likely to develop the disease. It is assumed that the curve of liability has a normal distribution in both the general population and in relatives (fig. 34) but the curve for relatives is shifted to the right. The point on the curves above which all individuals are affected is the *threshold*. In the general population the proportion above the threshold is the population incidence and among relatives the proportion above the threshold is the familial incidence. This model has been used to explain the familial incidence of the comparatively common disorders already mentioned i.e. certain congenital abnormalities, peptic ulcer, diabetes mellitus, etc. In conditions in which the inheritance is believed to be multifactorial there are several consequences of such a model. The incidence will be greatest among the relatives of more severely affected individuals because presumably they are more extreme deviants along the curve of liability. Thus in cleft lip with or without cleft palate the proportion of affected relatives (sibs and children) is roughly 6 per cent (1 in 16) when the index patient has double hare lip and cleft palate, but only 2·5 per cent (1 in 40) if he only has a single hare lip. By similar reasoning it would also be expected that the incidence among sibs born subsequent to the index case would be greater the more affected relatives there were in the family. In spina bifida (p. 131) for example, after the birth of a single affected child the incidence among subsequent sibs is approximately 4 per cent, but 10 per cent after the birth of two affected children and evidence suggests the risk is higher still if another close relative is also affected. This is quite different from the situation in unifactorial traits where the risk in subsequent sibs remains constant irrespective of the number of affected individuals in the family already (e.g. 1 in 4 for an autosomal recessive trait).

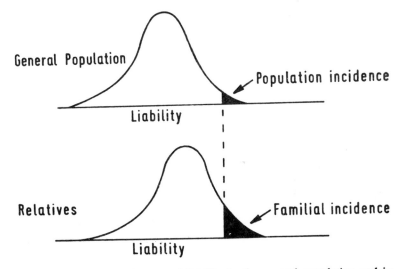

Figure 34. Hypothetical curve of liability in the general population and in relatives for a hereditary disorder in which the genetic predisposition is multifactorial.

Finally in multifactorial inheritance it follows that when there is a sex difference in the population incidence, the relatives of an affected individual of the less frequently affected sex will be more often affected. The explanation in this case is probably that the curve of liability has the same distribution in both sexes but that of the less frequently affected sex is shifted to the left so that they are more extreme (compared with the normal members of their own sex) when they are affected. This is exemplified in the condition of congenital pyloric stenosis, a condition which is characterized by persistent vomiting after feeds and was invariably fatal until Ramstedt introduced a curative operation in 1912. Carter has made a careful study of the condition among the various relatives of affected individuals including the offspring of persons who themselves were affected and successfully treated in childhood. Though pyloric stenosis is five times commoner in boys than girls, the proportions of affected relatives of male index patients are 5·5 per cent for sons and 2·4 per cent for daughters but 19·4 per cent for sons and 7·3 per cent for daughters when the index patient is a female.

HERITABILITY

Though it is not possible to assess the individual's liability to a particular disease it is possible to estimate how much of the aetiology can be ascribed to genetic factors as opposed to environmental factors. This is the so-called *heritability* which may be defined as the proportion of the total variation of a character which can be attributed to genetic factors. It is therefore expressed as a percentage and often abbreviated to the symbol ' h^2 '. The greater the value for the heritability the greater the contribution of genetic factors to aetiology. The heritability can be calculated from the known incidences of a particular condition in relatives and in the general population. Estimates of heritability for some common diseases are given in table XIII. Thus genetic factors would seem to be much more important in the aetiology of congenital pyloric stenosis than in peptic ulcer. However it should be realized that estimates of heritability depend on the degree of resemblance between relatives and this may in part be due to sharing of a common environment. It is therefore important to derive estimates from different kinds of relatives, and not sibs alone, and to measure the frequency of the condition in relatives reared or living apart and in unrelated individuals living together, such as spouses, in order to assess the possible effects of common environmental factors.

So far familial predisposition to disease has been interpreted in terms of liability and it has been assumed that liability is normally distributed. This is somewhat of an abstraction and for this reason other models have been proposed. Space does not permit an adequate treatment of these various models which are largely based on mathematical reasoning. The interested reader is referred to recent articles where the problem has been discussed in more detail (Falconer, 1965, 1967; Carter, 1969; Edwards, 1969).

One interesting result of the liability model is that the concordance in twins depends on the population frequency of the disease as well as on the heritability (Smith, 1970). With a high heritability the concordance rate in identical twins may be quite low. For example, in club foot, the incidence of which is 1 in 1000 and the heritability is about 70 per cent, the concordance rate in identical twins is only 33 per cent.

Table XIII. *Estimates of heritability for various disorders affecting man*

Disorder	Incidence (%)	Heritability
Asthma	4	80
Schizophrenia	1–2	80
Cleft lip ± cleft palate	0·1	76
Pyloric stenosis (congenital)	0·3	75
Diabetes mellitus: early onset	0·2	75
late onset	2–3	35
Ankylosing spondylitis	0·2	70
Dislocation of hip (congenital)	0·07	70
Club foot (congenital)	0·1	68
Coronary artery disease	3	65
Hypertension (essential)	5	62
Anencephaly and spina bifida	0·5	60
Peptic ulcer	4	37
Congenital heart disease (all types)	0·5	35

The determination of familial incidence not only gives us an idea of the contribution of genetic factors in aetiology but is essential for genetic counselling. Further, the investigation of the genetics of common disorders should not stop at the stage of the multifactorial hypothesis. The next step is to identify the contribution of individual gene loci to aetiology.

116 ELEMENTS OF MEDICAL GENETICS

FURTHER READING

Carter, C. O. (1969). Genetics of common disorders. *Br. med. Bull.* **25**(1), 52–57.

Edwards, J. H. (1969). Familial predisposition in man. *Br. med. Bull.* **25**(1), 58–64.

Emery, A. E. H. and Walton, J. N. (1967). The genetics of muscular dystrophy. *Prog. med. Genet* **5**, 116–145.

Falconer, D. S. (1965). The inheritance of liability to certain diseases estimated from the incidence among relatives. *Ann. hum. Genet.* **29**, 51–76.

Falconer, D. S. (1967). The inheritance of liability to diseases with variable age of onset, with particular reference to diabetes mellitus. *Ann. hum. Genet.* **31**, 1–20.

Fraser, F. C. (1963). Taking the family history. *Am. J. Med.* **34**, 585–593.

McKusick, V. A. (1964). *On the X Chromosome of Man.* Washington D.C.: American Institute of Biological Sciences.

McKusick, V. A. 1975). *Mendelian Inheritance in Man.* 4th ed. London : Johns Hopkins Univ. Press.

Morton, N. E., *et al.* (1970). Discontinuity and quasi-continuity: Alternative hypothesis of multifactorial inheritance. *Clin. Genet.* **1**, 81–94.

Smith, C. (1970). Heritability of liability and concordance in monozygous twins. *Ann. hum. Genet.* **34**, 85–91.

Stern, C. (1957). The problem of complete Y-linkage in man. *Am. J. hum. Genet.* **9**, 147–166.

Stevenson, A. C. and Cheeseman, E. A. (1956). Heredity of deaf mutism with particular reference to Northern Ireland. *Ann. hum. Genet.* **20**, 177–231.

Taussig, L. M., Lobeck C. C., Agnese, P. A. S. *et al.* (1972). Fertility in males with cystic fibrosis. *New Eng. J. Med.* **287**, 586–589.

Whissell, D. Y., Hoag, M. S., Aggeler, P. M. *et al.* (1965). Hemophilia in a woman. *Am. J. Med.* **38**, 119–129

VII

Genetic Factors in Some Common Diseases

In general, only rare diseases are inherited in a simple manner; in common diseases, there is usually no simple pattern of inheritance. For example, in cancer of the breast, investigations have clearly shown that genetic factors undoubtedly play a part in causation but it would be impossible to explain these findings solely in terms of mendelian inheritance. Unifactorial or multifactorial inheritance is probably involved in the aetiology of many diseases but the picture is almost always complicated by environmental factors.

Susceptibility to pulmonary tuberculosis is inherited but only a small proportion of genetically predisposed persons actually develop the disease because nutritional state, general health, and exposure to infection are of greater importance than genetic predisposition. In peptic ulcer, genetic factors are also involved since the condition is twice as common among the sibs of patients as in the general population. However, it is quite clear that peptic ulceration is connected with stress and worry. Environmental factors are probably more important than genetic factors. It is true to say that it is uncommon for heredity or environment to be entirely responsible for any particular trait or disease. In most cases both factors are responsible though sometimes one may appear more important than the other (fig. 35). At one extreme we have diseases such as Down's syndrome or Duchenne muscular dystrophy which are exclusively genetic in origin and where the environment seems to play no direct part in aetiology. At the other extreme we have infectious diseases which are almost entirely the result of environmental factors. Between these extremes are such conditions as diabetes mellitus, hypertension, ischaemic heart disease, peptic ulcer, schizophrenia, certain cancers and congenital abnormalities in which both genetic and environmental factors are involved. These disorders are the subject of this chapter. The treatment here, of course, does not set out to be an exhaustive study of the genetics of these conditions but rather indicates *the ways in which investigators elucidate the role of genetic factors in common diseases.*

In attempting to understand the genetics of a particular condition, the investigator may approach the problem in a number of ways. He can study the incidence of the disease among relatives, compare the incidence in identical and non-identical twins, compare incidences in various racial groups, study the association of the disease with various other characteristics such as the blood-groups, and finally he may study pathological components of the disease in relatives, e.g. serum lipids among the relatives of patients with ischaemic heart disease. The study of animal analogues (diseases in animals which are analogous to diseases which occur in humans) may also be helpful. Each of these approaches will be illustrated with reference to a number of fairly common disorders.

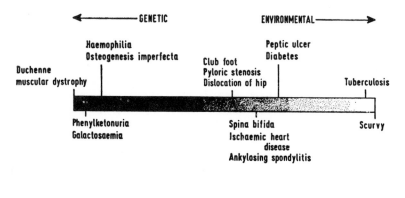

Figure 35. Human diseases represented as being on a spectrum ranging from those which are largely environmental in causation to those which are entirely genetic.

DIABETES MELLITUS

There are two clinically distinct forms of diabetes mellitus: a very severe form which comes on during childhood or in early adult life, and a much milder form which affects older people. The former can only be controlled by regular injections of insulin which must be maintained throughout the patient's life but the mild form usually responds simply to dietary restrictions. Diabetic women frequently have overweight babies and are more likely to have stillbirths and babies with certain congenital malformations. This is also true of some women who develop diabetes mellitus later on but at the time they are pregnant do not have clinical manifestations of the disease.

The evidence that diabetes mellitus is, at least in part, genetically determined comes mainly from studies of twins and from knowledge of the frequency of the disease among relatives of affected persons. Concerning data from twin studies it is necessary to add a word of caution. If both members of a pair of identical twins have the same trait this does not prove that the trait is hereditary. Since twins tend to share the same environment it is possible they will be exposed to the same hazards. For example, if one of them contracts a contagious disease such as impetigo, it is more than likely that the other will also become affected, but obviously impetigo is not hereditary. This difficulty can be partly resolved by comparing differences between non-identical and identical twin pairs on the assumption that both types of twins will have a tendency to share the same environment but whereas identical twins have identical genotypes, non-identical twins are no more similar genetically than brothers and sisters. If a trait is entirely genetically determined then, barring such rare events as chromosome non-disjunction in one twin, both members of a pair of identical twins will be similarly affected but non identical twins may differ. If a trait is entirely due to environmental factors, then differences between twins will be very much the same whether they are identical or non-identical.

Though all twins tend to share the same environment, it is probable that this is more likely in identical twins than it is in non-identical twins. Similarities between identical twins may thus reflect their shared environment as much as their identical genotypes. One way of getting round this difficulty would be to study differences between identical twins reared apart. If a particular trait is entirely genetically determined then whenever one identical twin is affected the other will also be affected even if they have been brought up in different environments. However, it is rare for identical twins to be separated from early childhood and so only a few published studies on such individuals exist. In one study of 19 pairs of identical twins reared separately the data clearly showed that each pair of twins differed little in height but differed considerably in their weight. These observations thus serve to verify that heredity plays a bigger part in determining stature than it does in determining weight.

Both members of a pair of twins are said to be *concordant* when either both are affected or neither is affected. The term *discordant* is used when only one member of a pair of twins is affected. In the case of diabetes mellitus one large survey showed that about 65 per cent of identical twins were concordant whereas only about 20 per cent of non-identical twins were concordant. At the time the study was made not all the twins had completed their life spans. It is probable that concordance rates would have been higher if all the twins had lived out their lives. Nevertheless the data certainly indicate that genetic factors are involved in diabetes mellitus but the fact that a significant proportion of the identical twins were discordant suggests that the genetic predisposition does not always manifest itself and that environmental influences must also be involved. Unfortunately no extensive studies have been made of diabetes in identical twins reared separately.

The Royal College of General Practitioners in London made a study of the first-degree relatives (parents, offspring and sibs) of 1307 diabetic patients and compared the results with the findings in first-degree relatives of a non-diabetic control group of 859 persons selected at random from the general population. With regard to the findings in the sibs of the propositi the results were very interesting. In the control group the proportion of those with a diabetic sib rose from about 0·3 per cent under age 30 to 2 per cent over age 70. In contrast, in the case of diabetics the proportion of affected sibs was about 5 per cent under age 30 and 3 per cent over age 70. This means that diabetics under 30 when diagnosed are about 15 times more likely to have an affected sib than healthy persons. In contrast, diabetics over 70 at diagnosis are only about 1·5 times as likely to have an affected sib. These results indicate that there is a strong genetic predisposition in those who develop the disease when young. In the elderly, diabetes mellitus is more the result of environmental factors, such as overeating.

Others have tackled the problem from a different angle. If the disease is due to a recessive gene (d) and an affected person (dd) has two unaffected parents, the parents must have the genotype Dd and it would be expected that 25 per cent (on the average) of their offspring should be affected. If one parent of an affected individual is a diabetic then the mating must be dd × Dd and 50 per cent of their offspring, should be affected. Finally if both parents are affected then all their offspring should be affected. The ratios of affected offspring in these three types of mating are therefore 25 : 50 : 100 or 1 : 2 : 4. Steinberg has obtained results which agree closely with these expected ratios based on the assumption that the disease is due to a recessive gene. From the data obtained in family studies it has been estimated that about 5 per cent of the general population must be homozygous for this gene. Nevertheless, surveys have shown that only about 1 per cent of the population has clinical signs of the disease. If diabetes mellitus is due to a recessive gene then the gene cannot be fully penetrant because only about 20 per cent of those who are presumed to be homozygous actually have the disease.

Some investigators who accept the idea that diabetes mellitus is due to a recessive gene have gone so far as to suggest that the severe childhood form of the disease represents the homozygous state whereas the milder form coming on later in life represents the heterozygous state. This view, however, is not shared by all investigators, and as we have seen, there is good evidence for believing that late onset diabetes is largely dependent on environmental factors.

Though some investigators believe that diabetes mellitus is inherited as an autosomal recessive trait others contend that the disease is the result of the action of many genes (multifactorial inheritance). In support of this idea it is pointed out that the incidence of the disease in parents and children (when correction is made for age) is as high as in sibs which is contrary to what would be expected if the disease were due to a recessive gene. Secondly, there is no clearcut separation between blood sugar levels after ingesting a given quantity of glucose, in relatives of diabetics and in control subjects. In both groups there is a continuous distribution from normal to abnormal values with no evidence of two ' humps ' (bimodality) which would be expected if the disease were due to a single gene. Evidence based upon the frequencies of diabetes mellitus in various relatives of affected individuals also suggests that the disease is inherited on a multifactorial basis.

Assuming multifactorial inheritance, Simpson and Smith have independently estimated the heritability to be about 75 per cent for early onset diabetes, but only 35 per cent for late onset diabetes.

An active field of investigation at present is the devising of tests for recognizing ' prediabetics '. These are persons who are genetically predisposed to developing diabetes but have not yet developed clinical manifestations of the disease. It seems likely that if such preclinical cases could be recognized then means might be found of preventing the disease from developing in later life. Investigations of individuals at risk (e.g. close relatives of affected individuals) are being undertaken at various centres and a reliable test for recognizing prediabetics may soon be available. Recent studies indicate that after ingesting a given dose of glucose the amount of insulin in the blood is abnormally high in at least some prediabetics. Vallance-Owen has shown that plasma albumin from patients with diabetes, and also from some prediabetics has more antagonism to insulin than normal individuals. To date these seem the most encouraging methods of detecting prediabetics.

HYPERTENSION

Patients with hypertension fall into two groups. In one of these the onset is usually in early adult life and is secondary to certain kidney diseases or abnormalities of certain endocrine glands. This form of hypertension is referred to as *secondary* hypertension and is rather uncommon. In the second group of patients there is no obvious cause for the disease, which usually begins in middle age. This form of the disease is referred to as *essential* hypertension and is much more common than secondary hypertension. The following discussion is concerned only with essential hypertension. It is generally agreed that genetic factors are important in the aetiology of essential hypertension for it has been shown that there is a high concordance in identical twins, but authorities differ as to the exact nature of these genetic factors. In essence there are two schools of thought.

On the one hand there are those who consider that blood pressure levels are distributed continuously in the population and people with hypertension merely represent one extreme of the distribution curve. They consider that blood pressure, like stature, results from the action of many genes. The evidence presented in favour of this concept is that if blood pressure measurements are made on a large enough number of people the results are normally distributed and show no evidence of any bimodality. It is also argued that blood pressure is the result of many different factors such as pulse rate, calibre of blood vessels, and so on and consequently it seems more logical that multifactorial inheritance should be the cause.

The other school of thought considers that essential hypertension is due to a single dominant gene. Evidence in favour of this idea has been presented by Platt. He argued that if essential hypertension is a disorder of middle age resulting from the action of a dominant gene it would be expected that the sibs of hypertensive patients would segregate into two groups: those who inherited the disorder and those who did not. He collected blood pressure readings of 252 sibs of persons known to have hypertension. He chose all his cases from the age group 45–60 in order to exclude, as far as possible, cases of secondary hypertension. He found that the blood pressure values of the sibs were not normally distributed but had a bimodal distribution with two peaks corresponding to blood pressures of 130 and 160 mm mercury (fig. 36). This suggests that those with values of about 130 had inherited the normal gene whereas those with values around 160 had inherited the gene for hypertension.

Evidence in favour of this idea has been presented by Morrison and Morris. They recorded the blood pressure of 302 symptomless London busmen aged 45–60 and found that the blood pressure readings were normally distributed. But when the same men were classified according to the longevity of their parents quite a different

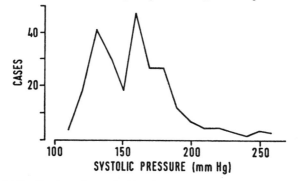

Figure 36. Distribution of systolic blood pressures in 252 sibs of persons aged 45 to 60 with hypertension. (After R. Platt, 1959, *Lancet* **2**, 57 with permission.)

result was obtained. Essential hypertension, especially if untreated, is a serious disease and frequently leads to death in middle age. Realizing this fact Morrison and Morris divided the parents of their busmen into those who died in middle age (40–64) and those who survived past the age of 65 on the assumption that this would give a crude subdivision into one group with more hypertension and another group with less hypertension. They found that the blood pressure values of busmen whose parents had lived to 65 or over were normally distributed and did not increase with age (fig. 37). However, in the group of busmen whose parents died in middle age, the blood pressure values showed a bimodal distribution with one peak at 140 and another at 175 mm mercury. In this group, blood pressure gradually increased with age.

Much of the controversy between the two schools of thought concerning the hereditary nature of hypertension revolves around the definition of bimodality. Critics of the single gene theory claim that what others have interpreted as bimodality are merely irregularities in the distribution curve and are of no significance. They point out that in small samples the distribution curve of heights may show small dips and irregularities but everyone agrees that this trait is controlled by numerous genes. If a large enough sample is taken, such as was done by the British during World War II when the heights of 91,163 recruits were recorded, then the resultant distribution curve has no irregularities.

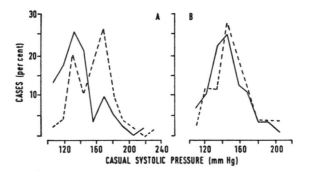

Figure 37. Distribution of casual systolic blood pressures in bus drivers aged 45–54 (continuous line) and 55–60 (interrupted line)—A, one or both parents died in middle age; B, both parents living to old age. (After Morrison, S. L. and Morris, J. N., 1959, *Lancet* 2, 865, with permission.)

It is probable that a more definite answer to the question of hereditary factors in hypertension will only be found when prospective studies are undertaken. As an example, it would be very informative if, in say 20 years' time, we were to compare Platt's two apparently different groups of sibs of hypertensive patients. If the bimodality in the distribution of blood pressure readings in the two groups were maintained then this would be good evidence that the disease is due to a single gene. Another point worth considering is that if hypertension is due to a single gene then according to the ' one gene-one polypeptide ' concept it would be expected that there is a specific primary biochemical abnormality which causes hypertension. So far a biochemical abnormality has not been detected. In recent years, through selective breeding experiments, hypertensive strains of rabbits, rats, and chickens have been developed. Biochemical investigations of these animals might provide a clue to the possible existence of a biochemical abnormality in human hypertension. It has been reported that hypertension is more frequent on the island of Tiree than on the mainland of Scotland. The interpretation of this finding in terms of aetiology is not clear but the study of this island community may throw more light on the cause of hypertension.

ISCHAEMIC HEART DISEASE

Atherosclerosis, with consequent narrowing of the coronary arteries producing ischaemic heart disease or ' coronary thrombosis ', is due in part to the deposition of lipid in the walls of the blood vessels. This is part of the natural ageing processes. However, the condition may occur prematurely leading to death in the third to fifth decades of life. One variety of early onset ischaemic heart disease is familial hypercholesterolaemia which is inherited as an autosomal dominant trait. (*see* Nevin & Slack, 1968). This accounts for only a small fraction of early onset ischaemic heart disease. Other cases are associated with some other disease such as diabetes mellitus. However, the majority of cases are not inherited in any simple way and are not associated with any other disease process. The general opinion is that in the majority of affected individuals the condition is multifactorial with a heritability of about 65 per cent. The risk to first degree relatives of an affected individual is on average six times the population incidence, the latter being about 15 per 1000 in males with onset before age 55, and 10 per 1000 in females with onset before 65.

PEPTIC ULCER

Peptic ulcers are of two kinds, gastric and duodenal, depending on whether the ulceration involves the lining of the stomach or the duodenum. In the individual case it may not be possible to say whether the lesion is in the stomach or the duodenum without a full clinical investigation including an X-ray examination. For this reason, and for the purposes of convenience, the two conditions are often lumped together. But this is probably not justified for it is possible that, as in the case of diabetes mellitus, we are dealing with two different diseases with different aetiologies. Gastric ulcer, for example, is more common in the lower social classes whereas duodenal ulcer is more frequent in the executive classes which suggests that different environmental factors are involved in the aetiologies of the two conditions. Heredity plays a part in the aetiology of both gastric and duodenal ulceration. The evidence comes from three sources: the frequency of ulcers among relatives of affected persons, twin studies, and blood-group studies.

Doll and his colleagues have shown that gastric and duodenal ulcers are twice as common among first-degree relatives of affected persons as in the general population and the type of ulcer tends to be the same in both the patient and his affected relative. It could be argued that the increased risk in close relatives may merely reflect a common family environment. The results of a recent extensive study in twins throws some light on the problem. Out of 29 identical twin pairs selected because one twin was affected, it was found that in 12 pairs the other twin was also affected. However, in the case of non-identical twin pairs of the same sex, in only 10 out of 46 were both affected. In other words the concordance in identical twins was roughly twice the concordance in non-identical twins which suggests the operation of genetic factors. But inasmuch as the concordance in identical twins was only about 41 per cent this means that environmental factors must also play an important part in aetiology.

Several studies in the last few years have shown that certain diseases are associated with particular blood groups more frequently than would be expected by chance. These observations suggest a causal relationship between a particular disease and the blood group with which it is associated. It is assumed that since the blood groups are inherited so genetic factors must play a part in the causation of the particular diseases with which they are associated. The best documented example of such an association is that of duodenal ulcer and blood-group O (fig. 38). This does not mean that all persons with blood-group O will develop a duodenal ulcer but merely that their risk of having a duodenal ulcer is greater than in persons with other blood groups. It has been calculated that persons with blood-group O are about 40 per cent more liable to duodenal ulcer than persons with blood-groups A, B, or AB. Gastric ulcer is also associated with blood-group O but the association is not so strong as in the case of duodenal ulcer. The association of blood-group O and duodenal ulcer has been found in Europeans, Japanese, North American Negroes, and several other racial groups. The association therefore cannot be simply due to studies having been limited to a particular group of people with a high frequency of group O and a coincidental high susceptibility to duodenal ulcer.

It is important to distinguish between association and genetic linkage. In association two conditions appear in the same person more often than would be predicted by chance and this implies a causal connection between the two conditions. Genetic linkage, however, is concerned only with the arrangement of genes on the chromosomes (p. 51). Genes are linked when they are carried on the same chromosome pair, and an important point is that linkage is between *loci* and not with one particular allele at a locus. For example, it has been found that a rare syndrome consisting of absent patellae and abnormal nails (the nail-patella syndrome) is linked to the ABO blood-group locus. The nail-patella gene is transmitted with the A blood-group gene in some families, with the B blood-group gene in others, and with the O blood-group gene in yet other families. The nail-patella syndrome is not associated with a *specific* blood group. Association implies that the two conditions which are associated are in some way causally related. On the other hand conditions due to genes which are linked bear no causal relationship to each other. A particularly strong association is that between ankylosing spondylitis and the HL-A antigen W27.

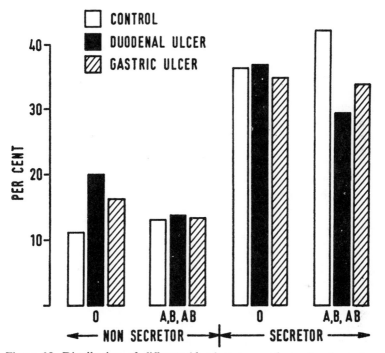

Figure 38. Distribution of different blood groups and secretor types in a control population and in patients with duodenal ulcer (1000 patients) and gastric ulcer (251 patients). (Data from C. A. Clarke and published with permission.)

Returning to the question of peptic ulcer, the manner in which the blood-group genes influence the lining of the stomach and duodenum is not known. Presumably, the integrity of the gastric and duodenal mucosae is under the control of several genes for peptic ulceration and is not only associated with blood-group O but also with secretor status. The ABO blood-group substances are secreted in the saliva and gastric juice of persons who carry the secretor gene (S). This gene is dominant to the non-secretor (s) gene. Persons homozygous for the non-secretors gene (ss) do not secrete ABO blood-group substances. It has been found that duodenal ulcers, and gastric ulcers to a lesser extent, are more common in persons who are non-secretors than persons who are secretors. In fact secretor status seems more important than a person's blood group in determining the likelihood of developing a peptic ulcer.

From the evidence presented so far it would seem reasonable to assume that peptic ulcer is due to a lack of some substance which in secretors and persons with blood groups other than O, protects the mucosal lining from ulceration. But this cannot be the entire answer because of all cases of peptic ulcer only about 25 per cent have blood group O and are non-secretors. Heredity must play a part in the aetiology of peptic ulcer but its effect is far outweighed by environmental factors. Peptic ulcer appears to be multifactorial in causation and the heritability has been estimated to be about 40 per cent, being higher for duodenal than for gastric ulcer.

SCHIZOPHRENIA

Schizophrenia is a psychotic illness with onset usually in early adult life. It is characterized by personality and emotional changes associated with a withdrawal from reality accompanied by hallucinations and delusions. It is the principal cause of chronic mental illness, affecting 1 per cent of the population. At present there are about 80,000 schizophrenic patients in mental hospitals in the United Kingdom. No *specific* biochemical abnormality has yet been identified in this disorder.

Most investigators agree that there is a genetic contribution to the aetiology of schizophrenia the nature and extent of this contribution however, is not clear, partly because of confusion concerning definitions, particularly in the use of the term *schizoid*. This refers to the schizophrenic-like disabilities often seen in relatives of schizophrenics. The problem arises because clinical criteria for clearly distinguishing the schizoid from normal personality are lacking. Problems of definition have been discussed in detail by Heston (1970). For the sake of simplicity we can regard the term schizoid as referring to a person with the fundamental symptoms of schizophrenia but in milder form. It has been estimated that roughly 4 per cent of the general population have schizophrenia or a schizoid disorder.

The results of several studies of the prevalence of schizophrenia and schizoid disorder among the relatives of schizophrenics are summarized in table XIV.

If the two conditions are considered together then almost 90 per cent of identical co-twins have one or other of these disorders as do approximately 50 per cent of first degree relatives. What interpretation can be put on these results? The simplest would be that schizophrenia and schizoid disorders are both inherited as an autosomal dominant trait with almost complete penetrance. The idea that schizophrenia and schizoid disorders represent a single genetic disease is supported by their clinical similarity, and the fact that both occur with almost equal frequency in identical co-twins of schizophrenics. If the two conditions are considered together, then the proportions of affected first degree relatives fits well with the hypothesis of autosomal dominant inheritance: 50 per cent of first

Table XIV. *Proportions (%) of first degree relatives of individuals with schizophrenia who are similarly affected or have a schizoid disorder (*age-corrected). Data compiled by Heston (1970)*

Relatives	Proportion (%) of relatives Schizophrenia*	Schizoid	Total schizophrenia + schizoid
Identical twin	46	41	87
Offspring (of 1 schizophrenic)	16	33	49
Sibs	14	32	46
Parents	9	35	44
Offspring (of 2 schizophrenics)	34	32	66
General population	1	3	4

(Copyright 1970 by the American Association for the Advancement of Science.)

degree relatives of an affected individual and 75 per cent of the offspring of two affected individuals. However, the proportions of affected more distant relatives do not fit the dominant hypothesis so well. Also, the high prevalence of schizophrenia in the general population must mean that if the condition is due to a single gene then the mutation rate must be unusually high (which is most unlikely) or that this is a heterogeneous condition (which is quite possible), or that there is some heterozygous advantage otherwise such a deleterious disorder would have been eliminated long ago by natural selection (p. 162). It has been demonstrated that schizophrenics have a higher than normal resistance to traumatic or surgical shock, to allergies in general and to a number of pharmacologically active substances such as histamine and insulin. It has been suggested that in historic times resistance to mass epidemics of diseases like smallpox and plague may have been a contributing factor to the present prevalence of schizophrenia. However this is speculative and there is no compelling supportive evidence. Schizophrenia is associated with many complex traits such as body build and intelligence, and many believe that environmental factors must play an important part in aetiology. Perhaps the prevalence among close relatives is partly due to their sharing a common environment. Some investigators now consider that schizophrenia may in fact be inherited on a multifactorial basis (see discussion in Slater & Cowie, 1971) with a heritability of about 80 per cent. However, with our present state of knowledge a firm statement on the nature of genetic factors in schizophrenia is not possible. Present research into the biochemistry of affected individuals and their relatives may well clarify the situation in the next few years.

CONGENITAL ABNORMALITIES

There are many recognized causes of congenital abnormalities. Some can be accounted for by infections contracted during pregnancy (rubella, toxoplasmosis and cytomegalovirus), others to drugs ingested during pregnancy (e.g. thalidomide and synthetic progestins), maternal exposure to radiation (which may cause microcephaly with mental retardation) or to maternal disease (e.g diabetes mellitus in the mother is associated with an increased risk of defects of the sacrum and lower limbs in the infant). Many other congenital abnormalities are due to single gene defects (e.g. the autosomal recessive form of microcephaly) or to recognized chromosome abnormalities (e.g. the autosomal trisomy syndromes). However several rare congenital defects, such as unilateral congenital amputation, do not appear to be genetic and have so far not been accounted for by any teratogenic agent and their cause remains obscure.

Certain fairly common congenital abnormalities are believed to be multifactorial in causation. These include spina bifida and anencephaly, the commoner forms of congenital heart disease, congenital pyloric stenosis, cleft lip and cleft palate, congenital club foot and congenital dislocation of the hip. Evidence in favour of multifactorial inheritance in these conditions has been assembled by Carter (1965). As was emphasized earlier, the investigation of the genetics of such disorders should not stop at the multifactorial hypothesis but should proceed to the identification of the contributions of individual loci. In the case of congenital dislocation of the hip some progress in this direction has already been made. The condition is predisposed to by a shallow acetabulum, the shape of which appears to be under polygenic control. The condition is also predisposed to by joint laxity which in the families of affected individuals appears to be inherited as an autosomal dominant trait. Further, experiments in animals have shown that joint laxity is influenced by oestrogen levels and this might therefore account for why congenital dislocation of the hip is commoner in females.

In spina bifida there is a defect in the vertebral column through which part of the spinal cord and meninges may protrude. Many children with milder degrees of this abnormality are helped by neurosurgery though their legs often remain paralysed. In anencephaly a part of the skull and brain fail to develop and the condition is incompatible with survival. These two conditions (spina bifida and anencephaly) are comparatively common affecting about one baby in every 200, and in some way are related because both abnormalities frequently occur in different members of the same family. No specific biochemical or chromosome defect has been identified in these conditions which are commoner in the offspring of older multiparous women and in the North West of England, Wales and Scotland than in South East England. Family studies have shown that the frequency among sibs is roughly 10 times greater than in the general population but on the other hand, identical twins are usually not concordant for these abnormalities. No unifying explanation has yet been found for these various observations. Perhaps most intriguing of all is the observation that the increased familial incidence occurs only in matrilineal descendants. This has led to the suggestion that spina bifida and anencephaly may be an example of cytoplasmic inheritance (Nance, 1969). Clearly much more work remains to be done if the causes of these congenital abnormalities are to be understood.

CANCER

A malignant tumour (=neoplasm) consists of an abnormal uncontrolled proliferation of cells with partial or often complete lack of organization. Malignant tumours invade surrounding tissues and often in the later stages of the disease, spread throughout the body (metastasize). The fact that the major criteria of malignancy are increased and uncontrolled growth, and since growth is under gene control, implies that genetic factors are involved in all cancers. However, in some cancers it seems that the *primary* cause is an abnormal gene (or genes) whereas in other cases the primary cause is environmental and the abnormal proliferation of cells is secondary to this. In man there is a rather rare condition known as polyposis coli. In this disease the whole of the large bowel is lined with numerous polyps. There is a high risk of carcinomatous change taking place in these polyps and without treatment more than 90 per cent of affected persons die from cancer of the bowel. Polyposis coli is inherited as an autosomal dominant trait and in this case the primary cause is an abnormal gene. Other unifactorial disorders associated with malignancy include neurofibromatosis or von Recklinghausen's disease (dominant) in which tumours of the peripheral and central nervous systems occur, xeroderma pigmentosum (recessive) in which skin cancers occur particularly in exposed areas of the skin, and retinoblastoma (some cases are dominant) in which malignant tumours of the retina occur. Other examples of rare unifactorial disorders associated with various neoplasms are given in table XV.

It should be borne in mind, however, that there are other cancers in which environmental factors are of primary importance and heredity seems to play no part in causation. This is true of ' industrial cancers ' which result from prolonged exposure to carcinogenic chemicals. Examples include cancer of the skin in tar workers, cancer of the bladder in analine dye workers, angiosarcoma of the liver in process workers making polyvinyl chloride (P.V.C.), and cancer of the lung in asbestos workers. In all these instances it would seem that the carcinogen evokes malignant change by altering the cell's metabolism, presumably by an effect on gene regulator mechanisms within the nucleus.

The distinction between primary genetic factors and exogenous factors in the aetiology of cancer is a useful one but is not always clear-cut. Some cancers are more common in certain races and this suggests a genetic cause. For instance skin cancer in Australian whites is much more common than in the native population, presumably because the melanin in the skin of the aborigines prevents the penetration of ultraviolet radiation. The prevalence of skin cancer in Australian whites is partly due to genetic factors (fair skin) and partly due to environmental factors. However, racial differences in the frequency of diseases do not necessarily imply that genetic factors are the cause of these differences. For example cancer of the penis is extremely rare in Jews suggesting that this is perhaps due to genetic factors. But it is also true that such cancers are extremely rare in males circumcised in infancy whether they are Jewish or not. The fact that cancer of the cervix is uncommon in married Jewish women is probably related to the practice of circumcision in the male because smegma, an oily substance which tends to accumulate under the foreskin in uncircumcised males is carcino-

Table XV. Some unifactorial disorders associated with neoplasia

	Clinical features	Neoplasia
Autosomal dominant		
Basal cell nevus syndrome	nevi, skeletal abnormalities, jaw cysts	basal cell carcinoma
Diaphyseal aclasis	multiple exostoses	sarcoma
Epiloia	mental retardation, epilepsy, adenoma sebaceum on the face	benign tumours of the retina, heart and kidney
Neurofibromatosis	café-au-lait spots, neurofibromata	neurofibromata, CNS tumours (e.g. acoustic neuroma)
Phaeochromocytoma and thyroid carcinoma syndrome	—	thyroid carcinoma
Polyposis coli	colonic polyps	colonic carcinoma
Retinoblastoma (bilateral)	—	retinoblastoma
Tylosis	thickening of palms and soles	oesophageal carcinoma in some families
Autosomal recessive		
Albinism	absence of pigmentation	skin carcinoma
Ataxia telangiectasia	ataxia, telangiectases, sino-pulmonary infections	lymphoreticuloses
Bloom's syndrome	dwarfism, light sensitive rash	leukaemia
Chediak-Higashi syndrome	partial albinism, photophobia, leucopenia, infections	lymphoma
Fanconi's anaemia	pancytopenia, congenital malformations, skin pigmentation	leukaemia
Xeroderma pigmentosum	freckle-like hypersensitivity to light	skin carcinoma
X-linked recessive		
Bruton's agammaglobulinaemia	bacterial infections, absence of plasma cells and Ig	lymphoreticuloses
Wiskott-Aldrich syndrome	eczema, thrombocytopenia, infections, bloody diarrhoea	lymphoreticuloses

genic. Breast cancer is six times more common in European than in Japanese women and though this may be a true racial difference and thus presumably a genetic difference in cancer proneness, it is also possible that it may only be a reflection of nursing habits and fertility.

In the majority of human cancers there is no clear-cut mode of inheritance nor is there any clearly defined environmental cause. Future work may reveal that in some of these cases the cause is a specific carcinogen and that heredity plays little part. In certain cancers genetic factors seem to play an important, but not exclusive, role in aetiology. Cancers of the stomach and breast seem to be of this type and we will now examine the evidence which has been brought forward for the existence of genetic factors in these diseases. The evidence comes from four sources: frequency of the disease in near relatives of affected persons, twin studies, blood-group studies, and the use of animal analogues.

The results of family and twin studies have shown that there is no proneness to cancers in general but only to specific cancers. Family studies have shown that the likelihood of a first-degree female relative of a patient with cancer of the breast also developing the same disease by the age of 85 is about 10 per cent. In appropriate control groups the likelihood is roughly 5 per cent. Since the age of onset of cancer of the breast shows considerable variation, the age of 85 was selected in calculating these risk figures to ensure that all those who were genetically predisposed had the chance to develop the disease if they were going to. Since few people reach the age of 85 the risk figure in the individual case is much less than those given above.

Similar studies in cancer of the stomach have shown that about 3 per cent of first-degree relatives are liable to develop the disease as against 1·5 per cent in controls. That the frequency of tumours of the type found in the propositi is greater among close relatives than in the general population suggests the operation of genetic factors in aetiology. But since the frequency in near relatives is small the expression of these factors must be greatly influenced by either the remainder of the individual's genes or the environment. There is some very good evidence that this is so. Macklin has found that cancer of the breast is less common in child-bearing controls than in the child-bearing relatives of patients with this disease, but the frequency in the child-bearing relatives is still less than in unrelated women who are childless. Child-bearing renders a woman somewhat immune to cancer of the breast. Similarly cancer of the stomach does not affect all sections of the community with equal frequency but is most common in the lower social classes, perhaps because of dietary factors.

Verschuer has made a careful study of cancer in identical and non-identical twins. He found that in the case of cancer of the breast and cancer of the uterus the concordance was slightly higher in identical twins. In the case of cancer of the stomach the difference in concordance between identical and non-identical twins was much greater. Three out of 11 (27 per cent) identical twins were concordant. This is further evidence that genetic factors are involved in the aetiology of cancer of the stomach but the fact that most of the identical twins were discordant (73 per cent) emphasizes the importance of environmental factors.

We mentioned earlier the genetic implications of finding an association of a particular disease with a specific blood group. The first carefully controlled study of this kind was by Aird and his colleagues in 1953, who studied cancer of the stomach. It was known that cancer of the stomach was slightly more common in the North than in the South of England but no really satisfactory explanation had been found for this. Aird and his colleagues argued that since blood group O is more common in the North of England perhaps cancer of the stomach and blood group O might be associated. In order to test this hypothesis they compared the frequencies of different blood groups in the general population with the frequencies in patients with cancer of the stomach. To their surprise they found an association not with blood group O but with blood group A. The geographical distribution still remains unexplained.

The use of animals with diseases comparable to certain diseases in man (animal analogues) has provided an extremely useful tool for medical research. This is especially so in the field of genetics for we can carry out breeding experiments in affected animals and from the results draw conclusions regarding the genetics of comparable diseases in man. Examples of such animal analogues include haemophilia in dogs, muscular dystrophy and leukaemia in particular strains of mice, congenital dislocation of the hip in German shepherd dogs, and recently phenylketonuria in monkeys. With regard to malignant tumours, a few breeds of dog such as Retrievers, are particularly susceptible, whereas other breeds, Pekingese and Chows, have a low cancer proneness. Particularly valuable have been studies of tumours in some strains of rabbit and fowl. But by far the most informative studies have come from investigations in mice. Certain inbred strains of mice have been developed in which 90 per cent or more of the individuals develop a particular type of tumour. The A (albino) Bittner strain is especially prone to develop tumours of the lung and breast; the C3H strain is particularly prone to develop breast tumours as well as tumours of the liver; the C58 strain is prone to develop leukaemia. Breeding experiments with mice have shown that cancer proneness is influenced by environmental factors. In strains with a high incidence of breast tumours, the frequency of these tumours is reduced by dietary restrictions and increased by high temperature.

Of particular interest has been the work of Bittner, who showed that the proneness to develop breast tumours in certain strains of mice depends on a combination of genetic factors as well as a ' milk agent '. In high incidence strains both genetic proneness and milk agent are involved, but in some low incidence strains there is no milk agent. The milk agent has been shown to be a virus which is usually transmitted by the mother's milk but may also be transmitted by the father's sperm. By using foster-mothers of cancer-free strains to suckle newborn mice from strains with a high cancer proneness it is possible to reduce the incidence of breast cancers from 100 per cent to less than 50 per cent. Alternatively it is possible to increase the incidence in cancer-free strains by suckling the newborn mice with foster-mothers from high cancer-prone strains. Other examples of virus induced tumours include the Rous sarcoma in fowls, Shope papilloma and myxoma in rabbits, and the Lucké kidney cancer in frogs. There is some evidence that certain viruses may be oncogenic (tumour forming) in man but such investigations are hampered by the lack of an experimental animal in which suspected viruses may be grown. Recent work on human breast cancer has in fact revealed virus-like particles morphologically indistinguishable from the Bittner agent of mice. These particles can be identified in breast milk particularly from women who have a family history of breast cancer. If breast cancer is a viral-induced disease transmitted by mother's milk then breast feeding by mothers with a family history of breast cancer is best discouraged (Borden, 1974). It seems likely that in some cancers of man there may be genetic proneness as well as a viral agent. It is also possible that the viral agent might behave as do certain so-called ' temperate ' bacteriophage. These phage are integrated into the host bacterial cell, where they are called prophage and their presence might be extremely difficult to demonstrate. However, on exposure to ultraviolet light, X-irradiation, or certain chemicals, including carcinogens, the phage particles multiply and burst out of the host cell and can then infect other cells. The real interest in a causative viral agent is that one might be able to produce a vaccine against a specific cancer and this would be of particular use in persons known to be genetically predisposed.

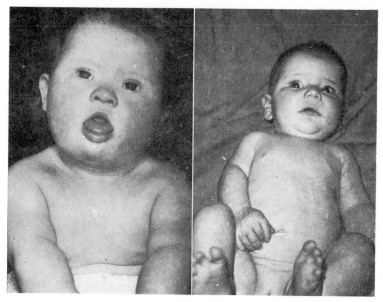

Plate 1. Down's syndrome.
Plate 2. Ellis-van Creveld syndrome; note the polydactyly.

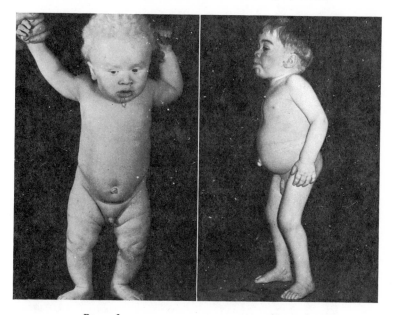

Plate 3. Albinism in a Negro child. (*By courtesy of Dr V. A. McKusick.*)
Plate 4. Hurler's syndrome. The protuberant abdomen is due to enlargement
of the liver and spleen.

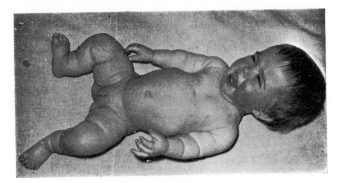

PLATE 5
Achondroplasia.

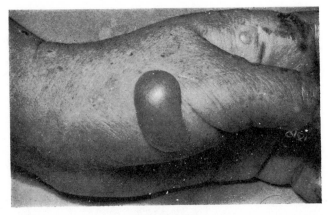

PLATE 6
Porphyria variegata; skin lesions on the hand.

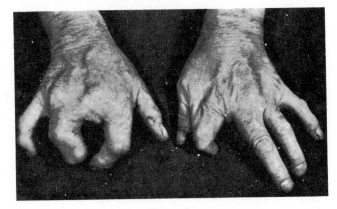

PLATE 7
Ectrodactyly (lobster claw deformity).

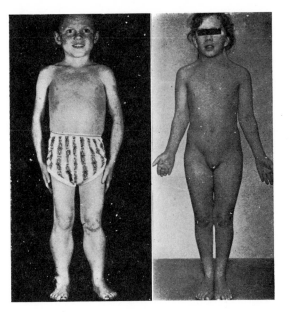

PLATE 8   PLATE 9

Plate 8. Duchenne muscular dystrophy; note the enlarged calves and wasting
of the thigh muscles.

Plate 9. Turner's syndrome; note the increased carrying angle at the elbow
and webbing of the neck.

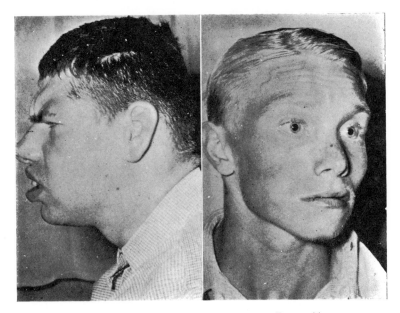

PLATE 10   PLATE 11

Plate 10. Microcephaly.

Plate 11. Phenylketonuria; note the fair complexion.

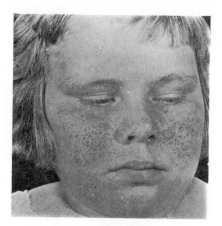

PLATE 12
Epiloia (tuberous sclerosis).

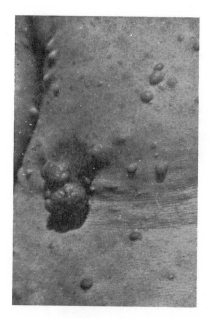

PLATE 13
Neurofibromata on the trunk in von Recklinghausen's
disease (neurofibromatosis).

Finally, recent work has provided biochemical evidence of the interaction of genotype and environmental carcinogens at least in the case of cancer of the lung. It appears that individuals differ in their ability to induce the enzyme aryl hydrocarbon hydroxylase (AHH) in the presence of certain polycyclic hydrocarbons (constituents of tobacco smoke) which are then converted to substances which produce cancer. Induction of AHH activity is due to the expression of two alleles at a single gene locus and about 10 per cent of individuals are homozygous for the ' high inducer ' gene. These individuals it seems, are at greater risk of developing cancer of the lung should they smoke (Kellermann et al., 1973). The determination of AHH inducibility, which can be determined on peripheral blood leucocytes, may be a way of identifying a high risk group in the population.

FURTHER READING

Aird, I., Bentall, H. H. and Roberts, J. A. F. (1953). A relationship between cancer of the stomach and the ABO blood-groups. *Br. Med. J.* 1, 799–801.

Borden, E. C. (1974). Viruses and breast cancer: implications of mouse and human studies. *Hopkins med. J.* 134, 66-76.

Carter, C. O. (1965). The inheritance of common congenital malformations. *Prog. med. Genet.* 4, 59–84.

Clarke, C. A. (1961). Blood groups and disease. *Prog. med. Genet.* 1, 81–119.

Detweiler, D. K. (1964). Genetic aspects of cardiovascular diseases in animals. *Circulation,* 30, 114–127.

Edwards, J. H. (1965). The meaning of the associations between blood groups and disease. *Ann. hum. Genet.* 29, 77–83.

Emery, A. E. H. and Lawrence, J. S. (1967). Genetics of ankylosing spondylitis. *J. med. Genet.* 4, 239–244.

Fedrick, J. (1970). Anencephalus: variation with maternal age, parity, social class and region in England, Scotland and Wales. *Ann. hum. Genet.* 34, 31–38.

Hawthorne, V. M., Gillis, C. R., Lorimer, A. R., Cavert, F. R. and Walker, T. J. (1969). Blood pressure in a Scottish island community. *Br. med. J.* 4, 651–654.

Heston, L. L. (1970). The genetics of schizophrenic and schizoid disease. *Science, N.Y.* 167, 249–256.

Huxley, J. (1958). *Biological Aspects of Cancer.* London: Allen and Unwin.

Huxley, J., Mayer, E., Osmond, H. *et al.* (1964). Schizophrenia as a genetic morphism, *Nature, Lond.* 204, 220–221.

Kellermann, G., Shaw, C. R. and Luyten-Kellermann, M. (1973). Aryl hydrocarbon hydroxylase inducibility and bronchogenic carcinoma. *New Engl. J. Med.* 289, 934-937.

Knudson, A. G., Strong, L. C. and Anderson, D. E. (1973). Heredity and cancer in man. *Prog. med. Genet.* 9, 113–158.

Laurence, K. M., Carter, C. O. and David, P. A. (1968). Major C.N.S. malformations in S Wales. *Br. J. prev. soc. Med.* 22, 146–160.

Lynch, H. T. (1969). Genetic factors in carcinoma. *Med. Clins N. Am.* 53(4), 923–939.

Macklin, M. T. (1959). Comparison of the number of breast-cancer deaths observed in relatives of breast-cancer patients and the number expected on the basis of mortality rates. *J. natn. Cancer Inst.* **22**, 927–951.

McConnell, R. B. (1966). *The Genetics of Gastro-intestinal Disorders.* London: Oxford University Press.

McKusick, V. A. (1964). A genetical view of cardiovascular disease. *Circulation*, **30**, 326–357.

Miller, J. R. and Yasuda, M. (1975). Environmental factors in the aetiology of congenital malformations in man. In *Modern Trends in Human Genetics.* Vol. 2. Ed. Emery, A. E. H. pp. 308-336. London: Butterworths.

Morrison, S. L. and Morris, J. N. (1959). Epidemiological observations on high blood-pressure without evident cause. *Lancet,* **2**, 864–870.

Nance, W. E. (1969). Anencephaly and spina bifida: a possible example of cytoplasmic inheritance in man. *Nature, Lond.* **224**, 373–375.

Nevin, N. C. and Slack, J. (1968). Hyperlipidaemic xanthomatosis. *J. med. Genet.* **5**, 9-28.

Pickering, G. W. (1961). *The Nature of Essential Hypertension.* London: Churchill.

Platt, R. (1964). The natural history and epidemiology of essential hypertension. *Practitioner,* **193**, 5–13.

Report of a working party appointed by the College of General Practitioners (1965). The family history of diabetes. *Br. med. J.* **1**, 960–962.

Rosenbloom, A. L. (1970). Insulin responses of children with chemical diabetes mellitus. *New Engl. J. Med.* **282**, 1228–1231.

Simpson, N. E. (1964). Multifactorial inheritance, a possible hypothesis for diabetes. *Diabetes,* **13**, 462–471.

Slack, J. (1969). Risks of ischaemic heart-disease in familial hyperlipoproteinaemic states. *Lancet,* **2**, 1380–1382.

Slack, J. and Evans, K. A. (1966). The increased risk of death from ischaemic heart disease in first degree relatives of 121 men and 96 women with ischaemic heart disease *J. med. Genet.* **3**, 239–257.

Slater, E. and Cowie, V. (1971). *The Genetics of Mental Disorders.* Oxford University Press.

Steinberg, A. G. (1959). The genetics of diabetes: A review. *Ann. N.Y. Acad. Sci.* **82**, 197–207.

Vallance-Owen, J. (1964). Synalbumin insulin antagonism and diabetes. *Ciba Fdn Colloq. Endocr.* **15**, 217–234.

Wynne-Davis, R. (1970). The genetics of some common congenital malformations. In *Modern Trends in Human Genetics.* Vol. 1. Ed. Emery, A. E. H. pp. 316-338. London: Butterworths.

Wynne-Davies, R. (1973). *Heritable Disorders in Orthopaedic Practice.* Oxford: Blackwell.

VIII

Pharmacogenetics

The term pharmacogenetics was introduced by Vogel for the study of genetically determined variations that are revealed *solely* by the effects of drugs. Such a definition excludes those hereditary disorders in which symptoms may occur spontaneously but are often precipitated or aggravated by drugs. Nowadays many investigators also include these diseases within the sphere of pharmacogenetics. During the last few years some very important discoveries have been made concerning the role of hereditary factors in the response of microorganisms and insects to drugs. For example, investigations are being made into the cause of penicillin resistance in certain strains of bacteria, and resistance to DDT and organophosphorous insecticides in insects. This is an exciting field of research, and one which has immediate application in clinical medicine and public health.

Until recently individual and racial differences in response to drugs in man were considered a nuisance, but now such variability has become a challenge to the medical investigator. For many years it has been known that some individuals may be especially sensitive to the effects of a particular drug whereas others may be quite resistant. Such individual variations may be the result of factors which are not genetic. For example, both the young and the elderly are very sensitive to morphine and its derivatives, as are persons with liver disease. Such variations do not come within the scope of pharmacogenetics which is only concerned with *genetically* determined variations in drug response. Because of the major advances in this subject over the last few years many consider that pharmacogenetics has earned its right to be considered a separate branch of genetics.

GENETICS IN DRUG METABOLISM

The sequence of events which are involved when a drug is metabolized is usually as follows:

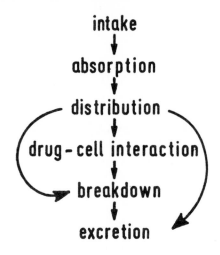

intake

absorption

distribution

drug - cell interaction

breakdown

excretion

Not all drugs are metabolized in this way, some for example are not broken down before being excreted. However, the metabolism of most drugs follows such a sequence. Thus, when taken by mouth, a drug is first absorbed from the gut and passes into the bloodstream, and so becomes distributed in the various tissues and tissue fluids. Only a small proportion of the total dose actually interacts with the cells to produce a specific pharmacological effect. Most of it is either broken down or excreted unchanged. The actual breakdown process, which takes place mainly in the liver, varies with different drugs. Some are completely oxidized to carbon dioxide which is exhaled. Others are excreted in various forms either via the kidneys into the urine, or via the liver into the bile and thence the faeces and many drugs undergo various biochemical transformations which increase their solubility so that they are more easily and readily excreted.

One important biochemical transformation is that of *conjugation* (= the union of two molecules) with the carbohydrate glucuronic acid, a process referred to as glucuronide conjugation. In the case of morphine and its derivatives, such as codeine, their elimination is almost entirely dependent on this process. Isoniazid, an important substance used in the treatment of tuberculosis, is 'acetylated' before it is excreted. This process involves the introduction of an acetyl group into the molecule.

Other drugs which are often acetylated before they are excreted include sulphonamides.

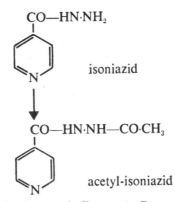

isoniazid

acetyl-isoniazid

In order to study the metabolism and effects of a particular drug the procedure usually adopted is to give a standard dose of the drug and then after a suitable time interval determine the response to the drug. This may involve measuring the amount circulating in the blood or making some other determination related to the rate at which the drug is metabolized. There is considerable variation in the way different individuals respond to certain drugs and the variability in response may be *continuous* or *discontinuous* (fig. 39). If a test is carried out on a large number of subjects and their responses are plotted, in continuous variation the results form a bell-shaped or unimodal distribution, but in discontinuous variation the curve is bimodal or sometimes trimodal. A unimodal distribution implies that the metabolism of the drug in question is under the control of many genes (p. 111) and the analysis of genetic factors in such cases is extremely complicated. In this discussion we will limit ourselves to those drugs the response to which is discontinuous, for in these cases the metabolism of the drug is under monogenic control. For example, if the normal metabolism of a drug is controlled by a dominant gene R and if some people are unable to metabolize the drug because they are homozygous for a recessive gene r, there will be three classes of individuals: RR, Rr, and rr. If the responses of RR and Rr are indistinguishable then a bimodal distribution will result. If RR and Rr are distinguishable then a trimodal distribution will result, each peak or mode representing a different phenotype (fig. 39).

GENETIC VARIATIONS REVEALED SOLELY BY THE EFFECTS OF DRUGS

Among the best-known examples of drugs which have been responsible for revealing genetic variability are hydrogen peroxide, isoniazid, succinylcholine, primaquine, certain anticoagulant drugs and anaesthetic agents.

In 1946 Takahara, a Japanese otorhinolaryngologist, treated an 11-year-old girl for a gangrenous lesion in her mouth. The infected tissue was excised and hydrogen peroxide was poured on the wound for sterilization. Normally with this treatment the blood oozing from the wound remains bright red and there is frothing. But Takahara observed that the blood which came in contact with the peroxide turned brownish-black and no bubbles formed. Takahara suggested that the patient's red cells might be deficient in the enzyme catalase

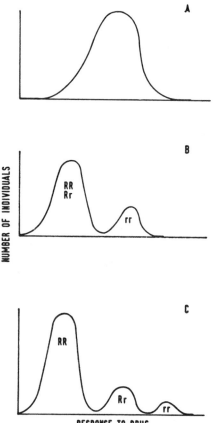

Figure 39. Various types of response to different drugs. A, Continuous variation, multifactorial control of drug metabolism; B and C, Discontinuous variation, monogenic control of drug metabolism.

which breaks down hydrogen peroxide into water and oxygen. He argued that if this enzyme were absent then hydrogen peroxide would not be broken down, there would therefore be no frothing, and the haemoglobin would be oxidized into methaemoglobin which is brownish-black in colour.

Subsequent studies showed that this condition is in fact due to lack of catalase and it has therefore been called acatalasia. Investigations of this girl's family and other families have shown that acatalasia is a rare recessive trait. Measurements of blood catalase activity have distinguished three classes of persons: those homozygous for the normal gene with normal levels of enzyme, those homozygous for the acatalasia gene with no enzyme in their blood, and heterozygous individuals with intermediate levels of enzyme. Acatalasia is not limited to Japan but has since been described in other parts of the world. Only about a half of those with acatalasia have oral sepsis, many have no symptoms at all and are perfectly healthy.

Isoniazid is one of the most important drugs used in the treatment of tuberculosis. Much work has been done on the metabolism of this drug. It has been shown that isoniazid is rapidly absorbed from the gut, resulting in an initial high blood level which is slowly reduced as the drug is inactivated and excreted. With regard to the metabolism of isoniazid two classes of persons can be clearly distinguished: rapid and slow inactivators. In the former, blood levels of the drug fall rapidly after an oral dose, in the latter, blood levels remain high for some time. Family studies have shown that slow inactivators of isoniazid are homozygous for an autosomal recessive gene while rapid inactivators are homozygous for a dominant gene. Heterozygotes are immediate with regard to the rapidity with which they inactivate the drug. The implication in these studies is that the rapid inactivator produces an enzyme which inactivates isoniazid but that this enzyme is absent in slow inactivators. In the United States and Europe about 50 per cent of the population are slow inactivators.

In some individuals isoniazid causes toxic symptoms such as polyneuritis. It might be predicted that since blood levels remain higher for longer periods of time in slow inactivators, toxic symptoms might be commoner in such individuals, and there is evidence which suggests that this is so. One would also expect that patients with tuberculosis who are treated with isoniazid might benefit more if they are slow inactivators than if they are rapid inactivators. However, this does not seem to be the case. Isoniazid inactivation phenotype does not seem to influence the response to treatment.

Phenelzine, a drug used in the treatment of depressive illness, has a molecular configuration similar to isoniazid. Not all patients respond to phenelzine and interestingly it may be possible to predict which patients will respond by their ability to inactivate isoniazid. Recent studies suggest that *slow* inactivators of isoniazid respond better to phenelzine than fast inactivators (Johnstone & Marsh, 1973). Similarly with hydralazine and sulphasalazine toxic side effects are more likely in slow inactivators of isoniazid.

Curare is a plant extract which has been prepared by certain tribes of South American Indians for many years. It produces profound muscular paralysis but with no loss of sensation and the Indians apply to the tips of their arrows when they are hunting. Medically curare has been used in surgical operations because of the muscular relaxation which it produces. Succinylcholine (*syn*: suxamethonium) is another drug which also produces muscular relaxation, though by a different mechanism from curare. This drug has an advantage over curare in that its action is only short-lived. The muscles of respiration are paralysed as well as the rest of the skeletal musculature, and consequently breathing stops for a short period, usually two or three minutes, after an injection of succinylcholine has been given. During this period of respiratory arrest (apnoea) the anaesthetist maintains respirations by artificial means. However, in about one patient in every 2000 the period of apnoea is very much prolonged and may last an hour or more. In such cases the apnoea can be corrected by a transfusion of blood taken from a normal person, otherwise the anaesthetist has to maintain the respirations until the effects of the drug have worn off. Succinylcholine is normally destroyed in the body by the enzyme pseudocholinesterase which is present in the blood plasma. In patients who are highly sensitive to succinylcholine the plasma pseudocholinesterase in their blood is abnormal and does not destroy the drug at a normal rate. In some very rare cases there is no enzyme. Family studies have shown that succinylcholine-sensitivity is inherited as an autosomal recessive trait.

A refined method of studying plasma pseudocholinesterase in the blood involves determining the percentage inhibition of the enzyme by the local anaesthetic dibucaine (*syn*: cinchocaine). The result is termed the dibucaine number. The frequency distribution of dibucaine number values in families with succinylcholine-sensitive individuals, gives a trimodal curve. The three modes represent the normal homozygotes, the heterozygotes, and the affected homozygotes. Experimental evidence clearly indicates that there are at least two different forms of plasma pseudocholinesterase: the one in the normal homozygote and the one in the affected homozygote. The two enzymes differ not only in the way in which they are inhibited by dibucaine (the enzyme in the affected homozygote being less inhibited) but also in their enzyme kinetics, the normal enzyme being more efficient than the abnormal enzyme in destroying acetylcholine and other choline esters. Extracts from solanaceous plants including the potato, have an effect similar to that of dibucaine in inhibiting plasma pseudocholinesterase, but the significance of this finding in terms of natural selection in human populations is difficult to assess.

For many years quinine was the drug of choice in the treatment of malaria but although it has been very effective in acute attacks it is not very effective in preventing relapses. In 1926 primaquine was introduced and proved to be much better than quinine in preventing relapses. Since then several other substances chemically similar to primaquine have been used. However, it was not long after primaquine was introduced that some people were found to be sensitive to the drug. The drug could be taken for a few days with no apparent ill effects, and then suddenly the patient would begin to pass very dark, often black, urine. Jaundice developed and the red-cell count and haemoglobin concentration gradually fell as the red blood cells were destroyed. The patient usually recovered from such a haemolytic episode but occasionally the destruction of the red cells was so massive as to be fatal. The cause of primaquine sensitivity was subsequently shown to be due to a deficiency in the red cells of the enzyme glucose-6-phosphate dehydrogenase (G6PD). However, the precise mechanism whereby G6PD deficiency brings about haemolysis in the presence of primaquine is still not clearly understood. Persons with G6PD deficiency are sensitive not only to primaquine but to many other compounds as well, such as phenacetin, furadantin, certain sulphonamides and acetylsalicyclic acid (aspirin). The ingestion of moth balls (naphthalene) may also lead to a haemolytic crisis in sensitive individuals and a deficiency of G6PD has been demonstrated in persons who develop haemolytic crises after eating fava beans (favism). Family sudies have shown that G6PD deficiency is inherited as an X-linked recessive trait. Red-cell G6PD deficiency is much commoner in negroes than Caucasians but in affected Negroes the enzyme activity in their *white cells* is normal whereas it is greatly reduced in most affected Caucasian males.

The coumarin anticoagulant drugs are used in the treatment of myocardial infarction to prevent the blood from clotting. Recent observations have suggested that there is discontinuous variation in the response of patients taking these drugs. In this case there is not an increased sensitivity but an increased *resistance* to the effects of the drug. For example, a patient has been described who required 20 times the usual dose in order to maintain adequate anticoagulation. This resistance appears to be transmitted as an autosomal dominant trait. Incidentally related substances have been used as a rat poison but recently resistant strains have been recognised. It seems the latter include more grass in their diet and the increased resistance is at least partly the result of increased intake of vitamin K from grass which counteracts the anticoagulant.

Recently the phenomenon of ' malignant hyperpyrexia ', a rare complication of anaesthesia, has been recognized to be genetic. Susceptible individuals develop hyperthermia, with temperatures as high as 42·3°C (108°F) and often with muscle rigidity, during anaesthesia usually when halothane is used as the anaesthetic agent and succinylcholine for intubation. If not recognized early and treated with vigorous cooling the patients often dies. The cause of the condition is not known but it appears to be inherited as a rare (roughly 1 in 10,000) autosomal dominant trait. Individuals who are genetically predisposed to developing malignant hyperpyrexia often have a raised serum level of creatine kinase and in families of affected individuals those at risk may be screened for in this way. However, a more accurate prediction of an individual's susceptibility to hyperpyrexia is possible by demonstrating an increased sensitivity to halothane, succinylcholine and caffeine of muscle biopsy specimens *in vitro*. The basic defect in this disorder appears to be a reduced uptake and binding of calcium ions to the sarcoplasmic reticulum (Moulds & Denborough, 1974). A patient known or suspected of having malignant hyperpyrexia can undergo surgery provided that precipitating anaesthetic agents are avoided. Should hyperpyrexia develop during surgery it can be treated by intravenous procaine or procainamide.

Phenylbutazone is used in the treatment of the more severe forms of arthritis. The metabolism of this drug differs from the examples discussed so far as it appears to be under polygenic control (Whittaker & Price Evans, 1970), though it is very likely that it is not unique in this regard. Recent work indicates that individuals who are relatively slow in metabolizing phenylbutazone are most likely to develop drug-associated toxic side effects such as hypoplastic anaemia.

HEREDITARY DISORDERS WITH ALTERED DRUG RESPONSE

It was pointed out at the beginning of this chapter that not all investigators include hereditary disorders with altered drug response within the sphere of pharmacogenetics. However, since it is a subject of immense importance in medical practice and touches on both genetics and pharmacology it is perhaps best discussed at this point.

Porphyria variegata is a condition which is usually inherited as an autosomal dominant trait. Some affected individuals have skin lesions—particularly on exposed surfaces—others have attacks of severe abdominal pain, muscular paralysis, and even mental disturbances. During an acute attack the patient may die. It has become recognized during the last few years that in persons genetically predisposed to porphyria, an acute attack may be precipitated by barbiturates. In parts of South Africa, where as many as 1 per cent of the population have porphyria, the possibility that any particular patient may have the disease and therefore be liable to an acute exacerbation if given barbiturates is a very real problem. Fortunately in Europe and the United States porphyria is much less common than in South Africa. Similar precautions have to be borne in mind in several other hereditary disorders in which severe exacerbations may be provoked by a particular drug. In G6PD deficiency, as we have seen already, the administration of sulphonamides to an affected person may result in severe haemolysis. Since G6PD deficiency is rare in most Caucasians but affects about 10 per cent of Negro males, sulphonamides, primaquine, and other sensitizing drugs have to be administered with caution to Negroes. Of course in a person *known* to be G6PD deficient such drugs would be absolutely contraindicated. Sulphonamides may also cause severe haemolysis in individuals with certain haemoglobinopathies. This is true in persons with haemoglobin H (a haemoglobin which consists entirely of beta-polypeptide chains) or haemoglobin Zürich which was first described in members of a Swiss family in 1962. But these are very rare conditions and in terms of numbers are much less of a problem than porphyria and G6PD deficiency.

In the treatment of congestive heart failure a number of drugs have been introduced during the last few years which have a diuretic effect. These drugs increase the excretion of water and consequently reduced the amount of oedema fluid. The most important of these diuretics is chlorothiazide which has been widely used because of its effectiveness and because it can be taken by mouth. However, not long after its discovery in 1957 it was realized that in persons with gout, the drug could cause serious side effects. Gout is a hereditary disorder associated with a raised serum level of uric acid. In genetically predisposed individuals attacks often follow dietary excesses which lead to an elevation in the serum uric acid. Chlorothiazide has a similar effect and this is particularly unfortunate because persons with gout often have hypertension and may develop congestive heart failure later in life. The genetics of gout is still not clearly understood. Some believe that the disease is inherited as a sex-influenced autosomal dominant trait, but recent work suggests it may be multifactorial. Since chlorothiazide raises the serum level of uric acid in genetically predisposed individuals the drug has been used in order to detect preclinical cases of the disease: persons genetically predisposed to the disease but who do not have symptoms. Unfortunately the results so far have not been very encouraging.

In the Crigler-Najjar syndrome the abnormal response to a drug has been used to detect carriers of this disease. This syndrome is characterized by severe nonhaemolytic jaundice often associated with cerebral disturbances. The jaundice appears on the first or second day after birth and persists throughout life. Affected children often die in infancy. The condition is inherited as an autosomal recessive trait, the heterozygote being perfectly healthy. The basic defect appears to be the inability of the liver to conjugate bilirubin with glucuronides due to a deficiency of the enzyme glucuronyl transferase. When drugs which normally undergo glucuronide conjugation (such as salicylates) are given to affected patients it is possible to show that they are unable to conjugate these substances. Defective salicylate conjugation has also been demonstrated in some carriers of this disease and the test has been used to identify such carriers.

The abnormal response to particular drugs in certain hereditary diseases has not only found application in the recognition of preclinical cases and carriers of these diseases but may also find use in differentiating between diseases which appear to be similar on clinical grounds but may be genetically different. In this regard some evidence suggests that it may be possible to differentiate between the various forms of depressive illnesses by their response to certain anti-depressant drugs. If this proves to be true, it would provide a very important tool for genetic studies of these diseases. The local application of corticosteroids (such as dexamethasone) and the measurement of subsequent changes in intraocular pressure may prove a useful means of studying the genetics of glaucoma and for detecting preclinical cases of this disease.

What is the evolutionary significance of these genetic variations in response to certain drugs? Man has been exposed to these drugs for no more than a few decades yet there is no doubt that mutant genes conferring abnormal responses to these drugs arose many thousands of years ago. As we shall see in the next chapter in the case of G6PD deficiency there is evidence which suggests that a deficiency of this enzyme may confer some protection against one form of malaria. But with regard to the other examples of hereditary variations in response to drugs we have very little idea as to their significance in relation to natural selection. Extracts of potatoes, tobacco leaves, and the foliage and roots of tomatoes are known to inhibit plasma pseudocholinesterase. A mutation which resulted in an enzyme not so inhibited might confer selective value under conditions where such foods were in abundance. It is possible that in the past, some metabolic variations may have conferred selective advantages under certain dietary conditions. Another possibility is that some might have conferred resistance to particular infections. However, at present we really have very little evidence on which to base these ideas. Some strains of rabbits are known to inactivate isoniazid rapidly whereas others do so slowly, and several other examples are known of animals with genetically determined variations in response to particular drugs. Observations on such animals under various experimental conditions might throw some light on these problems but so far the field is almost unexplored.

FURTHER READING

Armaly, M. F. (1968). Genetic factors related to glaucoma. *Ann. N.Y. Acad. Sci.* **151**, 861–875.

Childs, B. Sidbury, J. B. and Migeon, C. J. (1959). Glucuronic acid conjugation by patients with familial non-hemolytic jaundice and their relatives. *Paediatrics, Springfield,* **23**, 903–913.

Evans, D. A. P. (1969). Pharmacogenetics. In *Selected Topics in Medical Genetics.* Ed. Clarke, C. A., pp. 69–109. London: Oxford University Press.

Evans, D. A. P., Manley, K. A. and McKusick, V. A. (1960). Genetic control of isoniazid metabolism in man. *Br. med. J.* **2**, 485–491.

Isaacs, H., and Barlow, M. B. (1973). Malignant hyperpyrexia. *J. Neurol. Neurosurg. Psychiat.* **36**, 228–243.

Johnstone, E. C. and Marsh, W. (1973). Acetylator status and response to phenelzine in depressed patients. *Lancet,* **1**, 567–570.

Lehmann, H. and Liddell, J. (1964). Genetical variants of human serum pseudo-cholinesterase. *Prog. med. Genet.* **3**, 75–105.

Lehmann, H., Silk, E. and Liddell, J. (1961). Pseudo-Cholinesterase. *Br. med. Bull.* **17**, 230–233.

Marks, P. A. and Banks, J. (1965). Drug-induced hemolytic anemias associated with glucose-6-phosphate dehydrogenase deficiency: a genetically heterogenous trait. *Ann. N.Y. Acad. Sci.* **123**, 198–206.

Moulds, R. F. W. and Denborough, M. A. (1974). Biochemical basis of malignant hyperpyrexia. *Brit. med. J.* **2**, 241–244.

O'Reilly, R. A., Aggeler, P. M., Hoag, M. S. *et al.* (1964). Hereditary transmission of exceptional resistance to coumarin anti-coagulant drugs. *New Engl. J. Med.* **271**, 809–815.

Pare, C. M. B., Rees, L. and Sainsbury, M. J. (1962). Differentiation of two genetically specific types of depression by the response to anti-depressants. *Lancet,* **2,** 1340–1343.

Porter, I. H., Boyer, S. H. and Watson-Williams, E. J. *et al.* (1964). Variation of glucose-6-phosphate dehydrogenase in different populations. *Lancet,* **1,** 895–899.

Takahara, S., Hamilton, H. B., Neel, J. V., Kobara, T. Y., Ogura, Y. and Nishimura, E. T. (1960). Hypocatalasemia: A new genetic carrier state. *J. clin. Invest.* **39,** 610–619.

Vesell, E. S. (1973). Advances in pharmacogenetics. *Prog. med. Genet.* **9,** 291–367.

Waldenström, J. and Haeger-Aronsen, B. (1967). The porphyrias: a genetic problem. *Prog. med. Genet.* **5,** 58–101.

Whittaker, J. A. and Price Evans, D. A. (1970). Genetic control of phenylbutazone metabolism in man. *Brit. med. J.* **4,** 323–328.

IX

Population Genetics and Natural Selection

So far we have considered the gene in terms of its physical and chemical nature and the manner in which it segregates within families. With this background it is now appropriate to discuss the behaviour of genes in populations. The study of genes in populations rather than in individuals is the province of that branch of human genetics known as population genetics. In this chapter we will discuss some of the problems facing population geneticists. These include answering such questions as: How can we determine the frequency of a gene in a population? What factors affect gene frequencies and why are some genes more common than others? What part does natural selection play in maintaining gene frequencies in man and what will be the effects of improvements in medical care on the frequency of harmful genes in human populations? Finally, what can we do to influence our own evolution?

GENE FREQUENCIES IN POPULATIONS

At first sight it might seem reasonable to expect that dominant traits would increase in the population at the expense of recessive ones. After all on the average three-quarters of the progeny of two heterozygotes will manifest the dominant trait, but only one-quarter will have the recessive trait. There will be three times as many progeny manifesting the dominant trait as manifest the recessive trait. But in a large randomly mating population where there are no disturbances by outside influences, dominants do not increase at the expense of recessives. In fact in such a population the relative proportions of the different genotypes remain constant from one generation to another. This is known as the *Hardy-Weinberg principle* which was put forward independently by an English mathematician, G. H. Hardy, and a German physician, W. Weinberg, in 1908. The Hardy-Weinberg principle is one of the most important in human genetics and so is worthy of some detailed consideration.

If we consider a system with two alleles 'A' and 'a', there will be three possible genotypes 'AA', 'Aa', and 'aa'. If we represent the proportion of 'A' genes in the population as p and the proportion of 'a' genes as q, then p plus q must represent the sum total of genes at this particular locus, that is $p+q=100$ per cent. Since gene frequencies are usually expressed as a fraction of unity, we therefore write $p+q=1$. If the two genes in the population are in the proportions p and q, the sperms and eggs will contain them in the same proportions and with random mating the various gametic combinations can be represented as (gene frequencies are given in parentheses):

Male gametes

		A (p)	a (q)
Female gametes	A(p)	AA (p^2)	Aa (pq)
	a(q)	Aa (pq)	aa (q^2)

The frequencies of the various offspring from such matings are therefore p^2 (AA), $2pq$ (Aa) and q^2 (aa).

Let us now consider that these progeny mate with each other. The frequency of the various matings can be represented as shown below:

Genotype frequency of male parent

		AA (p^2)	Aa $(2pq)$	aa (q^2)
Genotype frequency of female parent	AA (p^2)	p^4	$2p^3q$	p^2q^2
	Aa $(2pq)$	$2p^3q$	$4p^2q^2$	$2pq^3$
	aa (q^2)	p^2q^2	$2pq^3$	q^4

For example, the frequency of matings between persons with the genotypes ' aa ' and 'Aa ' is $2pq^3 + 2pq^3 = 4pq^3$. The frequency of the various types of *offspring* from these matings can be represented as:

Mating type	Frequency	Frequency of offspring		
		AA	Aa	aa
AA × AA	p^4	p^4	—	—
AA × Aa	$4p^3q$	$2p^3q$	$2p^3q$	—
Aa × Aa	$4p^2q^2$	p^2q^2	$2p^2q^2$	p^2q^2
AA × aa	$2p^2q^2$	—	$2p^2q^2$	—
Aa × aa	$4pq^3$	—	$2pq^3$	$2pq^3$
aa × aa	q^4	—	—	q^4

Total

$$
\begin{aligned}
&= p^2(p^2 + 2pq + q^2) + 2pq(p^2 + 2pq + q^2) + q^2(p^2 + 2pq + q^2) \\
&= \quad p^2(p+q)^2 \quad + \quad 2pq(p+q)^2 \quad + \quad q^2(p+q)^2 \\
&= \quad\quad p^2 \quad\quad + \quad\quad 2pq \quad\quad + \quad\quad q^2
\end{aligned}
$$

So we see from this that the *proportion* of the various genotypes is the same in the second generation as it was in the first generation. We could continue such calculations for many generations, but the result would always be the same: the relative proportions of the genotypes would remain constant from one generation to another, and would occur in the proportions $p^2 : 2pq : q^2$.

This analysis is more than an exercise in elementary algebra, because knowing the proportions of the various genotypes (p^2, $2pq$, q^2) it is possible to derive the frequency of the various genotypes in the population if we know the frequency of one of the homozygotes (usually the rarer). Thus, alkaptonuria affects about one child in every 1,000,000. Therefore:

$$q^2 = \tfrac{1}{1000000}$$
$$\text{therefore } q = \tfrac{1}{1000}$$
$$\text{but } \quad p = 1 - q$$
$$\text{therefore } p = 1 - \tfrac{1}{1000}$$
$$\simeq 1$$
$$\text{The frequency of carriers } = 2pq$$
$$= 2.1.\tfrac{1}{1000}$$
$$= \tfrac{1}{500}$$

This example also illustrates another important point which is that in the general population carriers are very much more common than affected individuals. We will refer to this point again later.

The Hardy-Weinberg principle as applied to human populations is probably only an approximation because the principle is only absolutely true under certain very specific conditions, and probably for any particular trait in man all these conditions are rarely satisfied. We will now consider the conditions under which the Hardy-Weinberg principle holds, and some of the factors which influence it.

FACTORS AFFECTING THE HARDY-WEINBERG PRINCIPLE

The Hardy-Weinberg principle is true only for large populations where there is no migration or selection against a particular genotype and where there is random mating, and a constant rate of mutation.

Let us first consider the effects of *mutation*. A mutation has been defined as a change in a gene and in man there are two ways of measuring the rate at which mutations occur. First, there is the *direct* method in which the proportion of new mutations is determined among the individuals of one generation. This method is only applicable for autosomal dominant traits which are always fully penetrant; that is, the characteristic is fully manifest in all heterozygotes. An example of this method is provided by a study of achondroplasia which was made in Denmark a few years ago. It was found that out of 94,075 children born in hospital in Copenhagen, 10 were achondroplastic dwarfs. Of these 10 cases, two had an affected parent and so were not the result of new mutations but had inherited the disease from their affected parents. Thus among 94,073 children of *unaffected* parents there were eight achondroplastics or one new case (mutation) in approximately 12,000 births. However, in each affected child the mutation could have occurred in either the gene supplied by the mother or in that supplied by the father. For this reason, the *mutation rate per gene* is 1 in 24,000 ($0 \cdot 000042$ or 42×10^{-6}). In other words the mutation rate is 42 mutations per million genes (or gametes) per generation.

The direct method of estimating mutation rates is not applicable to recessive traits since a mutation to a recessive gene will go unrecognized if the mutant gene is completely recessive and not manifest in the heterozygote. This is also true of X-linked recessive traits. The method is only applicable to severe dominant traits in which affected individuals rarely, if ever, have offspring so that each affected person is most probably the result of a new mutation.

If a dominant gene is not lethal but merely reduces fertility then the picture is complicated because the number of affected individuals in any one generation will be composed not only of those who are the result of fresh mutations but also of those who inherited the mutant gene from an affected parent. In order to avoid these difficulties in the case of autosomal dominant traits with reduced fertility, and in autosomal recessive and X-linked traits, a second, *indirect*, method is used to estimate mutation rates. In this method we have to resort to a little algebra.

If μ (Greek letter *mu*) is the mutation rate per gene per generation then the frequency of cases due to fresh mutations is not equal to μ but is equal to 2μ since a mutation may occur on a chromosome derived from either parent. Consequently the frequency of the condition (F) is equal to 2μ. But as we have seen already this is true only for lethal autosomal dominant traits. If the condition is not lethal but the reproductive fitness (f) is less than normal (100 per cent) then in each generation the number of cases eliminated

$$= (100 - f)F$$

In a state of equilibrium where the frequency of the condition does not change from generation to generation, then the number of cases arising as a result of new mutations must be equal to the number being eliminated because of reduced fitness. Thus

$$2\mu = F(100 - f)$$

and therefore

$$\mu = \tfrac{1}{2}F(100 - f)$$

It is customary to express normal fitness as unity, and reduced fitness as a proportion of unity, therefore

$$\mu = \tfrac{1}{2}F(1 - f)$$

Similarly it can be shown that for an autosomal recessive trait

$$\mu = F(1 - f)$$

and for an X-linked recessive trait

$$\mu = \tfrac{1}{3}F(1 - f)$$

The term $(1 - f)$ is sometimes referred to as the coefficient of selection (s) against the gene.

Let us now consider the example of an autosomal dominant trait with reduced fitness. Mørch in Denmark found that 457 unaffected sibs of achondroplastics had a total of 582 children, so it would be expected that if the 108 achondroplastics he studied had possessed normal fertility then they should have had 137·5 children $(108/457 \times 582)$. In fact they had only 27 children so that their reproductive fitness $(f) = 27/137 \cdot 5 = 0 \cdot 1963$. That is, for every 100 children produced by their normal sibs, the achondroplastics had 19·63. The frequency (F) of the condition was 10 cases in 94,075 births (p. 149), therefore

$$F = \frac{10}{94,075}$$

and

$$\mu = \tfrac{1}{2} \cdot \frac{10}{94,075} \; (1 - 0·1963)$$
$$= 0·0000427$$
$$= 42·7 \times 10^{-6}$$

Mørch's study of achondroplasia has been chosen because it illustrates the way in which mutation rate may be calculated. Recent work, however, indicates that the mutation rate for achondroplasia derived from this data is excessively high. Dr R. J. M. Gardner has summarised the findings of newborn surveys in Manchester, Uppsala, Jersey City and Edinburgh and found six mutant *true* achondroplastics out of a total of 234,000 births giving a mutation rate of $12·8 \times 10^{-6}$. It is possible that Mørch included in his study a number of cases which would not now be considered true achondroplasia.

The indirect method only gives an approximate estimate of the mutation rate because it depends on the assessment of biological fitness which is often very difficult to determine with any accuracy. Another complication is that some of our estimates for mutation rates for certain traits may be too high because clinically similar,

Table XVI. *Estimates of ' spontaneous ' mutation rates (per million genes per generation) for certain traits in man*

Trait	Mutation rate
Autosomal dominants:	
Achondroplasia	12
Retinoblastoma	20
Epiloia	10
Polyposis coli	20
Neurofibromatosis	100
Huntington's chorea	5
Myotonic dystrophy	12
Autosomal recessives:	
Albinism	28
Total colour blindness	28
Phenylketonuria	25
X-linked recessives:	
Haemophilia A	20–32
Duchenne muscular dystrophy	43–95

but genetically different, conditions have been lumped together (table XVI). This is certainly true of earlier estimates of the mutation rate for ' haemophilia '. It is now known that there are at least two biochemically distinct forms of this disease which are due to different genes situated at different loci on the X chromosome. In order to determine mutation rates with any accuracy it is necessary to know the exact type of condition being studied. Without very careful biochemical tests, as in the case of haemophilia, this is sometimes not possible.

Furthermore, if calculations are based on the incidence of a disorder in the population then clearly the estimated mutation rate will be different for different races if the disorder occurs with different incidences. The figures given for recessives in table XVI apply only to western Europe.

Finally the age of the parent may also influence the mutation rate. For example, mutation rates for some disorders increase with *maternal* age (e.g. Down's syndrome and Klinefelter's syndrome) whereas others are related to *paternal* age (Marfan's syndrome, achondroplasia, Apert's syndrome, myositis ossificans and possibly bilateral retinoblastoma). The reason for this is not known.

Returning now to the effect of mutation on the Hardy-Weinberg equilibrium. Unless the amount of radiation to which we are exposed increases considerably or a new and potent mutagen is introduced into our diets it is probable that the rate of mutation for any particular gene will remain fairly constant. However it should be remembered that the mutation rates usually quoted for such conditions as achondroplasia may be atypical. A fresh mutation has never been observed in any of the blood groups. Mutations of these traits are probably exceedingly rare. (The subject of mutation will be discussed further in chapter X.)

Random mating (panmixis) means that the particular genes carried by an individual do not influence his choice of mate. In the case of the ABO blood groups it is almost certain that there is random mating since even if one knew one's blood group it would hardly influence one's choice of partner. But this is not true for other traits such as intelligence or stature where the choice of a partner is certainly not random. When mating is not random it is referred to as *assortative mating*. Assortative mating tends to increase the porportion of homozygotes in the population, and inbreeding has the same effect. Inbreeding is a particularly important factor in small isolated populations, often referred to as *isolates*. In such isolates the members of the community are prevented from marrying outside their group because of religious (e.g. the Amish people and certain Jewish sects), political and cultural (e.g. the Finns) or geographical (e.g. the Hopi Indians of Arizona) factors. The increase in homozygosity which results from inbreeding is reflected in the number of severe recessive conditions which are often found in these communities.

The genetic study of isolates has proved very rewarding for it has led to the recognition of several new recessive diseases. For example, a new syndrome, the cartilage-hair hypoplasia syndrome (Mc Kusick's syndrome), has been discovered in the Amish in North America. In this condition affected persons are dwarfed due to hypoplasia of the cartilage in growing bones, and their scalp hair is sparse, fine, and light in colour. Studies of this same isolate have also led to the recognition in certain diseases, such as hydro-metrocolpos, of a genetic component not previously suspected. In hydrometrocolpos there is a transverse vaginal septum and the new-born female infant has an abdominal tumour which consists of a dilated vagina and uterus. The finding of multiple affected sibs in several families of this inbred isolate suggests that at least one form of this rare malformation is due to an autosomal recessive gene with manifestations only in females. The prevalence of certain hereditary diseases in particular racial groups (Damon, 1969) might be explained by a mutation having occurred in the past in a member of the group which, because of social or economic reasons, remained isolated from others and so retained the gene within the group. One of the original members of a small isolated population may by chance have carried an otherwise rare gene which thereafter, as a consequence of inbreeding, becomes disseminated throughout the population. This is referred to as the *founder effect*.

In small isolated populations there is another factor besides in-breeding which may disturb the Hardy-Weinberg equilibrium. This is referred to as *random genetic drift* (fig. 40). In large populations, variations in the number of children produced by individuals with different genotypes has no significant effect on gene frequencies. On the other hand, in a small population such variations may have a considerable effect on gene frequencies. Random genetic drift may lead to the establishment of neutral or even unfavourable characters in a population. We can imagine how it might occur. Either because of social or geographical factors a small group of individuals might become isolated from the general population. If in the general population there were two alleles 'A' and 'a', where 'a' is the rarer, then by chance it might happen that nearly everyone in the isolate has the 'A' gene but only one or two carry the 'a' gene. If the few people carrying the 'a' gene do not have children or they have children but by chance do not transmit this gene to their offspring then, barring a fresh mutation, in one generation the 'a' gene will have completely disappeared from the isolated population. In these circumstances it is said that the 'a' gene has become *extinguished* and the 'A' gene has become *fixed*. Whenever chance leads to fixation of one allele and extinction of the other, an irreversible situation is established. The speed with which random genetic drift occurs depends on the size of the population, being greatest in small populations where oscillations in gene frequencies may be considerable.

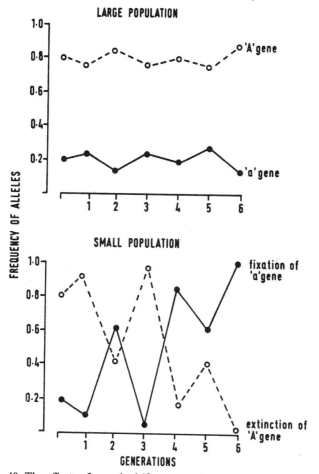

Figure 40. The effects of genetic drift on gene frequencies in large and small populations.

Table XVII. *Rare recessive disorders which are relatively common in certain groups of people*

Group	Disorder	Clinical features
Finns	Congenital nephrotic syndrome	oedema proteinuria susceptibility to infection
	Aspartylglycosaminuria	progressive mental and motor deterioration coarse features
	MULIBREY-nanism	MUscle, LIver, BRain and EYe involvement
	Congenital chloride diarrhoea	reduced Cl⁻ absorption diar- rhoea
Amish	Cartilage—hair hypoplasia	dwarfism fine, light coloured and sparse hair
	Ellis-van Creveld syndrome	dwarfism polydactyly congenital heart disease
Hopi and San Blas Indians	Albinism	lack of pigmentation
Ashkenazi Jews	Tay-Sachs' disease	progressive mental and motor deterioration, blindness
	Gaucher's disease	hepatosplenomegaly bone lesions skin pigmentation
	Dysautonomia	indifference to pain emotional lability lack of tears hyperhidrosis
Afrikaners	Sclerosteosis	increased stature syndactyly cranial nerve palsies

In large populations drift occurs slowly and oscillations in gene frequencies are only slight.

Random genetic drift has been evoked as a possible explanation for several observed differences in human blood groups. A particularly interesting one is that of the distribution of blood groups among North American Indians. The majority of North American Indians are blood-group O but among the Blood and Blackfeet

Indians blood-group A is particularly frequent. In fact, blood-group A is more common among these Indians than in any part of the world. It can be imagined that the immigrant ancestors of the American Indian brought all three (A, B, and O) blood groups with them from Asia but a small group of Indians became isolated and due to random genetic drift in this small isolate, blood-group A became very common. Random genetic drift might also explain abnormal blood-group frequencies in other small isolates such as the Dunkers, a religious sect in Pennsylvania. Similarly it might be the reason for the high frequency of an albino gene among the San Blas Indians of Panama, and a form of progressive muscle wasting (amyotrophic lateral sclerosis), believed to be genetically determined, which accounts for nearly 10 per cent of all adult deaths among people of the Marianas Islands but is extremely rare elsewhere in the world. Perhaps the high frequency of the Ellis-van Creveld syndrome (dwarfism, polydactyly, and congenital heart disease) among the Amish in Pennsylvania is also a result of random genetic drift. However before assuming that random genetic drift is the explanation for the high frequency of a particular gene in a population other factors should also be considered. For example, the high frequency (1 in 200) of albinism among the Hopi Indians of Arizona, is better explained by cultural selection rather than random genetic drift: albinos have been protected in the Hopi society and affected males have a sexual advantage over their normal peers.

The combination of founder effect coupled with isolation and inbreeding as well as genetic drift may all play a part in explaining the high frequency of rare recessive disorders in certain groups of people (table XVII).

It is perhaps obvious that migration would lead to changes in gene frequencies. Migrations of populations into new territories might result in contacts between diverse populations with resultant exchange of genes between these populations. Geneticists refer to this phenomenon as *gene flow*. The frequency of the gene for blood-group B is very high in Asia (over 25 per cent) but gradually decreases as one travels westward across Europe, until in Britain, France, and Scandinavia it is less than 10 per cent. Candela has explained this gradient as being the consequence of invasions by Mongoloids who pushed westward from about A.D. 500 until A.D. 1500. Miscegenation between the invaders and the native population, in which blood-group B is presumed to have been absent, led to the diffusion of the B gene from Asia across Europe. Gene flow is not the only possible explanation, however. It might also have been the result of some as yet unknown selective force which followed a similar geographic gradient. Gene flow alone certainly cannot explain the present blood-group frequencies among Amerindians. Blood-group O is very common in Indians from both North and South America but is rare in Asiatics, yet there is good evidence from other sources that the Amerindian is descended from Asiatic ancestors who migrated across the Bering Straits several thousands of years ago.

Knowing the frequency of the blood-group genes in Negroes in West Africa, in Caucasians, and in Negroes in the United States, it has been possible to estimate the amount of gene flow between Negroes and Caucasians in the United States. From such data it has been calculated that about 26 per cent of the total gene pool of the American Negro in Detroit is of Caucasian origin but only 4 per cent in Charleston, South Carolina. For obvious reasons gene flow has been almost exclusively from Caucasians into Negroes.

A very important factor which will disturb the Hardy-Weinberg equilibrium is *selection*. Selection forces operate by increasing or decreasing fitness. Fitness in the biological sense has a very special meaning. It is a measure of fertility and therefore of the contribution made to the genes of the succeeding generation. It may be defined as the number of offspring who reach the mean age at which the parent reproduced, so that infant deaths and stillbirths are excluded when calculating reproductive fitness.

Selection may operate on a gene at any time from conception into adult life. For example, from the point of view of selection a mutant gene is ' lethal' whether it interferes with embryogenesis and so causes an abortion, or whether it causes sterility in an otherwise normal person as in the testicular feminization syndrome.

Selection forces may be either natural or artificial. Natural selection occurs under natural conditions without the intervention of man. Artificial selection, on the other hand, is a direct consequence of man's intervention by introducing effective treatments for otherwise lethal conditions and limiting the reproduction of persons with hereditary defects. Artificial selection is not entirely a phenomenon of modern times for various eugenic measures have been practiced in the past, such as the castration of epileptics during the Middle Ages in Scotland.

In a state of equilibrium the rate at which a detrimental trait is produced by new mutations is balanced by the rate at which the trait is removed from the population by selection forces. Assuming that the mutation rate remains unchanged, then it would be expected that genes conferring greater biological fitness would tend to increase whereas those lowering biological fitness would tend to decrease.

This is true, but the situation is a little more complicated than it seems at first. It has been argued that if persons with serious hereditary diseases were sterilized then the frequency of such defects would be considerably reduced in future generations. There is no doubt that such measures would bring about a reduction in human suffering but they could never completely eradicate such diseases and in the case of rare recessive disorders it would take several generations to bring about any appreciable change in their frequency (fig. 41). The reasons for this are as follows. It can be shown that for a recessive trait

$$q = \sqrt{\mu/s}$$

and for a rare dominant trait

$$q = \mu/s$$

where q = gene frequency; μ = mutation rate, and s = coefficient of selection.

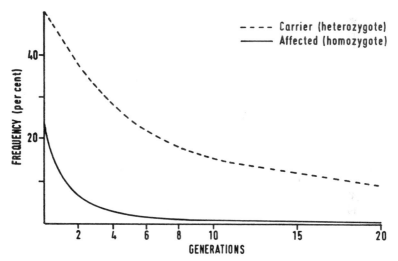

Figure 41. The effects of complete selection against a recessive trait. Before selection the frequency of homozygotes is taken to be 25 per cent and the frequency of heterozygotes to be 50 per cent. Note that it takes about five generations to reduce the frequency of the heterozygotes by half.

Obviously if fertility is reduced to zero (by sterilizing all affected persons), the coefficient of selection will be unity ($s = 1 - f$), and the ultimate frequency of a trait, irrespective of whether it is dominant or recessive, will depend on the mutation rate. That is, for a recessive trait the frequency of affected individuals will be $q^2 = \mu$; for a dominant trait the frequency of affected individuals will be approximately 2μ. Thus even if all affected persons were sterilized there would come a time when the frequency of the condition could be reduced no further.

In the case of a dominant trait the effect of sterilizing affected individuals would be immediate. In the case of a recessive trait the new equilibrium would be reached only very slowly (fig. 41). The reason for this difference is that in recessive conditions, most of the genes in the population are carried by perfectly healthy heterozygotes who would not be affected by such eugenic measures (table XVIII).

Table XVIII. *Approximate frequencies of affected homozygotes and heterozygotes of some recessive conditions*

Condition	Frequency of homozygotes (q^2)	Frequency of heterozygotes $(2pq)$	Consanguinity (%)
Alkaptonuria	1/1,000,000	1/500	25
Cystinuria	1/100,000	1/160	9
Albinism	1/20,000	1/70	5
Phenylketonuria	1/10,000	1/50	3
Fibrocystic disease	1/2,000	1/22	—
Sickle-cell anaemia (parts of Africa)	1/25	1/3	—

It can be shown that if there is complete selection against a recessive trait (all the homozygotes die or do not reproduce) then the number (n) of generations required to change the gene frequency from q_0 to $q_n = 1/q_n - 1/q_0$. Thus, if we take the case of a recessive condition which occurs with a frequency of 1 in 2000 births, and we were to sterilize all affected individuals then in order to reduce the frequency by half it would take over 500 years:

$$q_0 = \sqrt{\frac{1}{2000}} \simeq \frac{1}{45}$$

$$q_n = \sqrt{\frac{1}{4000}} \simeq \frac{1}{63}$$

so that in this illustration $n = 18$ generations. With rarer conditions it would take even longer. For example, if a condition occurs with a frequency of 1 in 20,000 births, then even with *complete* selection against the homozygote it would take over 1700 years to halve the frequency and this ignores the addition of new mutations. Selection against a recessive gene is extremely ineffective when the gene is rare and is most effective at intermediate gene frequencies. It is axiomatic that selection is most effective for common traits and ineffective for rare ones.

Another complication with regard to recessive traits is that with the advent of modern civilization the amount of inbreeding has gradually declined so that the frequency of affected homozygotes, on whom selection operates, has also diminished. It might therefore be expected that the frequencies of many recessive genes are probably lower than their equilibrium values and some may be increasing to new equilibria with higher values, but so slowly that the changes are imperceptible. On the other hand some recessive conditions, in which at one time the heterozygote may have had a selective advantage, may now be decreasing. We will discuss this in more detail later.

Selection against X-linked recessive genes resembles the effects of selection against autosomal dominant genes since X-linked recessives are manifest in hemizygous males, as are dominant traits. However a proportion of X-linked recessive genes are carried by heterozygous females who are phenotypically normal and thus not directly subject to selection. Hence selection against X-linked recessives is more effective than against autosomal recessives but less effective than against autosomal dominants. If selection were complete; that is, all carriers could be recognized and they all decided not to have any children, then the number of boys born with the disease could be reduced to the level of the mutation rate. If we could recognize all carriers (at present we can only recognize some of those who carry the more severe X-linked recessive conditions) and they all agreed to limit their families, the number of boys affected with such diseases as Duchenne muscular dystrophy would be reduced to a third.

Let us now consider the reverse condition where selection operating against a serious genetic disorder is relaxed so that more affected individuals reach adult life and can transmit the mutant gene to their offspring. This is the situation which can be expected in the case of a disease such as phenylketonuria where affected children no longer die or require institutionalization but can grow up into healthy adults if given correct treatment during childhood. The result will be that the frequency of the mutant gene will increase until a new equilibrium is reached with a much higher frequency of the deleterious gene in the population. If the treatment became available to all affected individuals simultaneously then in the case of a dominant gene the frequency of the deleterious gene would immediately increase then gradually level off at a new equilibrium value. Thus, if at one time all those with a serious autosomal dominant disorder died in childhood ($f=0$) then the frequency of those affected would be 2μ, but if improved treatment raised the fitness of affected individuals to 0·9 then the frequency of affected children in the next generation would increase to 2μ (from fresh mutations) *plus* $\frac{9}{10} \times 2\mu$ (survivors) which is $3 \cdot 8\mu$. In succeeding generations there would be $5 \cdot 4\mu$, $6 \cdot 9\mu$, $8 \cdot 2\mu$, and so on until equilibrium was eventually reached when the number affected can be calculated to be 20μ. The net result would be that the *proportion* of children who die will be less, but the *number* affected will be considerably greater and the actual number who die from the disease will remain unchanged. We have seen already that selection against a recessive gene is extremely ineffective when the gene is rare and is most effective at intermediate gene frequencies. This is also true if selection *favoured* a recessive gene. The response would be similar to that of a dominant gene though equilibrium would only be reached after a much longer period of time, because while the gene was rare it would be represented almost entirely in heterozygotes who would be unaffected by selection.

After the foregoing discussion of the effects of selection, it might be worthwhile to consider for a moment genes which have been considered to be neutral as regards their survival value.

The ability to taste phenylthiocarbamide (PTC) might be considered a neutral gene. About 70 per cent of Caucasians experience a very bitter taste if this substance is applied to the tongue, whereas the remaining 30 per cent find the substance tasteless. Family studies have shown that the ability to taste PTC is due to a dominant gene T, tasters having the genotype TT or Tt and non-tasters being tt. It is difficult to visualize how this particular characteristic could have any selective advantage, and for this reason it was considered a neutral gene. The genes for colour blindness and the ABO blood groups have also been considered neutral as regards selection. Nevertheless. Fisher has shown that for a gene to be neutral the balance of advantage between the gene and its allele must be very precise, and the chances of survival of such genes are small. In fact it is doubtful if any human trait is completely neutral as far as selection is concerned. The more we learn of the effects of genes the less likely it seems that any are entirely neutral. For instance recently an association has been found between the ability to taste PTC and certain types of thyroid disease, which raises the possibility that the ability to taste PTC and the metabolism of thyroxine and similar substances are related in some way and this may be of importance from the point of view of selection. We have seen that certain blood groups are associated with peptic ulcer and cancer of the stomach which indicates that the blood-group genes are not entirely neutral. In the case of colour blindness the situation is more speculative. It has been suggested that colour blindness might actually have been of advantage in primitive man since colour-blind persons are less confused by camouflage. Whatever the mechanism, colour blindness presumably had a selective advantage at one time in man's evolution.

GENETIC POLYMORPHISM

We have seen that for a recessive condition, the number of unaffected heterozygotes in the population is very large compared with the number of affected homozygotes. In general a very small increase in fertility of the carrier compared with the normal homozygote would easily balance a gene's selective disadvantage in the affected homozygote. For example, it can be calculated that in phenylketonuria an increase in fertility of only 1 per cent in the heterozygote would more than outweigh the loss of genes in affected children who die. This is because the small increase in fitness would be spread over a great many carriers in the general population. Of course, such a small increase in fertility would be very difficult to detect. In phenylketonuria there is no need to postulate any advantage in the heterozygote in order to maintain the present gene frequency because this could be maintained by rare mutations. By contrast, in conditions such as fibrocystic disease and sickle-cell anaemia affected homozygotes are so common that we either have to postulate that the genes responsible for these conditions have extremely high rates of mutation, which is very unlikely, or the high gene frequencies are maintained by a selective advantage in the heterozygote. Such *hybrid vigour* or *heterosis* has been recognized for many years by plant and animal breeders and the concept has now been introduced into human genetics.

In a large population if any genetic condition (excluding polygenic traits) occurs with a frequency of more than a few per cent this must be the result of a selective advantage in the heterozygote since the frequency of the condition could not be accounted for by mutation alone. This constitutes what is referred to as *genetic polymorphism* which may be defined as the occurrence together in the same habitat of two or more discontinuous forms of a species in such proportions that the rarest of them cannot be maintained merely by recurrent mutation (see Ford, 1960). There are two types of polymorphisms: balanced and transient. In a balanced polymorphism two or more

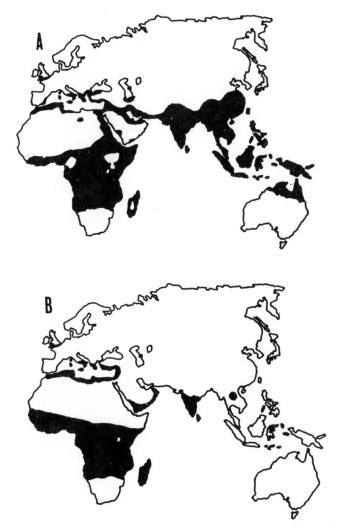

Figure 42. A. World distribution of falciparum malaria prior to 1930; B. World distribution of sickle-cell trait. (Data from A. C. Allison and published with permission.)

different forms are maintained by a balance of selective advantages and this usually arises when a heterozygote is favoured compared with either homozygote. The best example in man is the sickle-cell gene (fig. 42). In parts of Africa up to 4 per cent of the population are affected and about one person in three is a carrier. This situation must have arisen because of an advantage in the heterozygote. Sickle-cell anaemia is most frequent in regions with a high incidence of a particularly virulent form of malaria (falciparum malaria due to infection with *Plasmodium falciparum*) and it has been found that carriers of the sickle-cell gene are more resistant to infection by this organism than are normal persons. It appears that in heterozygotes, parasitization of an erythrocyte by *P. falciparum* substantially increases its probability to sickle and that once sickled, the parasitized cells are more effectively removed from the circulation by phagocytosis. This seems to be the mechanism whereby heterozygotes are at a selective advantage over normals.

Malaria not only causes early death but predisposes to considerable ill health. In a community in which malaria is endemic those who are more resistant to infection will not only survive better but will have a higher reproductive fitness. The increased fertility of the heterozygotes balances the elimination of sickle-cell genes through affected homozygotes. The American Negro no longer has the selective advantage of the heterozygote, since he is not exposed to malaria, and the result has been that the frequency of sickle-cell trait has gradually fallen until at present it is less than 10 per cent. In the American Negro the sickle-cell polymorphism is a *transient* one, because owing to a change in the environment the frequency of the sickle-cell gene is falling in each successive generation.

The classical example of a transient polymorphism in animals is seen in the case of the peppered moth (*Biston betularia*). The first black specimen was recorded in the North of England in 1850. toward the end of the industrial revolution. Because of its colouring the new variety blended better with the grimy surroundings in industrial regions than the original peppered form (fig. 43). Since then the black variety has gradually increased, at the expense of the peppered variety, as industrial pollution has extended. It should be remembered that in nature other mechanisms may also be responsible for determining the prevalence of a particular form. Predators often concentrate on one or a few common varieties of prey and tend to overlook the rarer forms even if they are obvious. Selection of this type has been referred to as *apostatic* because it involves the advantage of rare phenotypes which stand out from the norm. Apostatic selection accounts for the frequencies of certain forms of land snails.

Thalassaemia is a disease which occurs mainly in the Mediterranean area and in Asia (p. 37). In certain parts of Italy over 10 per cent of the population carry the thalassaemia gene which in the homozygous state causes a severe haemolytic anaemia which is usually fatal in early childhood. The high frequency of the thalassaemia gene must be the result of increased fitness of the heterozygotes. There is some evidence that the heterozygote may have had

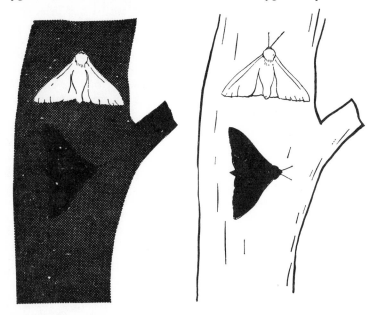

Figure 43. The peppered moth (*Biston betularia*). Typical and black varieties on different backgrounds.

an increased resistance to malaria. Since World War II, however, malaria has been largely eliminated from the Mediterranean so that whatever advantage the heterozygote may have enjoyed in the past no longer obtains and we may expect the gene frequency gradually to fall to a new equilibrium at a lower level.

Glucose-6-phosphate dehydrogenase (G6PD) deficiency is also found in Mediterranean countries, parts of Africa, and in Asia; the world distribution closely follows that of falciparum malaria. We have seen already that this enzyme deficiency may cause severe haemolytic anaemia in hemizygous affected males (p. 145). Evidence suggests that the high frequency of the G6PD deficiency gene in certain parts of the world is also due to increased resistance to malaria in heterozygous females. It seems clear that haemoglobin S and G6PD deficiency both offer a selective advantage to the carrier against potentially lethal falciparum malaria.

An interesting point worth considering in regard to geographic polymorphisms is the possibility of genetic regulatory mechanisms at the population level. That is, gene frequencies giving a high genetic load at one locus are often associated with those giving low genetic loads at other loci (Parsons). For example, among Kurdish Jews there is a high incidence of thalassaemia and G6PD deficiency but a low incidence of rhesus negative individuals, and in many parts of the world where malaria was endemic the frequency of rhesus negative individuals is often low. It has been suggested that such regulatory mechanisms have gradually evolved so that the over-all genetic load is never excessive.

Before leaving the subject of polymorphisms mention should be made of the serum proteins and certain other biochemical systems which can be used for the genetic description of populations since the allele frequencies of the traits vary in different populations. Human serum contains about 7 grams of protein per 100 ml. The protein consists mainly of albumins and globulins. In 1955, Smithies described a new method of separating serum proteins by electrophoresis in starch-gel. The details of the method need not concern us here, but in essence it consisted of placing a little serum in a small trough cut in a block of starch-gel and then passing an electric current through the starch-gel. By this means it is possible to resolve serum proteins into many different fractions some of which are under genetic control (fig. 44).

The serum protein fractions which are under genetic control include the haptoglobins (α-globulins) and the transferrins (β-globulins). The haptoglobins are globulins which contain a relatively high content of carbohydrate and have an affinity for haemoglobin. On starch-gel electrophoresis it is possible to recognize various types of haptoglobins, the three most common types being designated 1—1, 2—1, and 2—2. Family studies have shown that the three types are determined by a pair of allelic genes Hp^1 and Hp^2 (Hp^1Hp^1 = 1—1; Hp^1Hp^2 = 2—1; Hp^2Hp^2 = 2—2). There are several other alleles at the Hp locus but they are rare. The frequency of the Hp^1 gene varies in different populations. For example the frequency of Hp^1 exceeds 80 per cent in parts of Africa but is less than 20 per cent in Australian aborigines.

The transferrins are also globulins but they migrate somewhat faster than the haptoglobins. The transferrins carry plasma iron and release it in certain tissues such as the bone marrow. On starch-gel electrophoresis the transferrins lie between the albumin bands and the haptoglobins. Most sera contain only a single transferrin band designated TfC. However in certain populations several variants have been recognized some of which migrate faster (the B series) and others which migrate more slowly (the D series) than TfC. Apart from TfD, which occurs in certain negroes, most of the other variants are comparatively rare. It is believed that the different variants are determined by a series of alleles at the Tf locus. Other

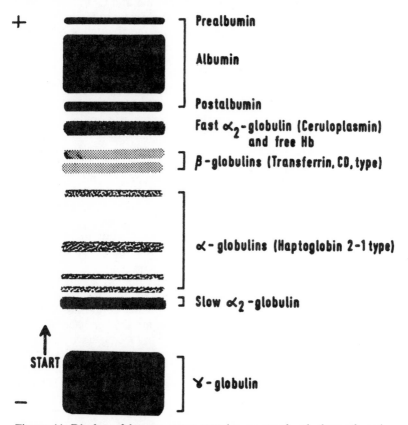

Figure 44. Display of human serum proteins on starch-gel electrophoresis.

polymorphisms which have frequently been used by anthropologists for defining populations include the ability to taste PTC (for example, non-tasters are much less frequent in Amerindians and Asiatics than in the rest of the world), colour vision, and the urinary excretion of beta-amino-isobutyric acid (BAIB). High excretors of BAIB are homozygous for a recessive gene whereas low excretors are either heterozygous or normal homozygotes. High excretors are particularly frequent among Amerindians and Africans. The selective advantages of these various genetic polymorphisms are completely unknown at the present time. The ability to taste PTC is not limited to man but has also been described in primates and even mice. The proportion of non-tasters in anthropoid apes is similar to that in humans and the fact that the polymorphism also occurs in mice raises the interesting question as to the nature of the factors responsible for maintaining this polymorphism across such a wide variety of species.

It has been shown from studies of isozyme and protein variability in *Drosophila*, that natural populations have polymorphisms at about 30 per cent of their structural gene loci and an average individual can be expected to be heterozygous for some 12 per cent of its structural loci. Professor Harris and his colleagues have also shown that a considerable amount of enzyme variation also occurs in human populations. He has stated that defective enzymes and proteins found in specific inherited diseases must be regarded simply as throughout the species and is in fact, one of its fundamental characteristics. In other words, inherited metabolic disease should be considered as merely one end of a spectrum of protein and enzyme variation. Since much variation would be expected to involve amino acid substitutions which alter the function of the resulting protein only slightly or not at all, it has been argued by some that most evolutionary changes in DNA and proteins are primarily due to neutral mutations and random genetic drift rather than to natural selection, so-called *non-Darwinian evolution*. Since much of the enzyme and protein variability found in natural populations does not *appear* to be associated with any obvious advantages in the heterozygote, it is difficult to account for these polymorphisms. However, as we have seen already, it is doubtful if any gene mutation is ever neutral in its effects and it seems more likely that evolutionary changes in DNA may well be attributable to natural selection but the nature of the selective forces has not yet been identified. Furthermore, strong selection on particular polymorphic loci may well affect the frequencies of alleles at adjacent *closely linked* loci.

Man's Future Evolution

Because of improved medical care we are prolonging the life of many individuals who would otherwise have died before reaching child-bearing age. The result will be an accumulation of ' bad ' genes in the population which would normally have been eliminated. This is the price we have to pay for being civilized. The question now arises,

'What can we do about this?' It would be unethical not to treat many of these conditions and there is no doubt that advances in medical treatment have helped to relieve an enormous amount of personal suffering. But if we are to continue treating such diseases we must also be prepared to face the consequences of having to deal with more affected persons in each succeeding generation. It has been argued that affected persons might be persuaded not to have children. Perhaps voluntary or even legislative sterilization might have to be considered in some cases, but it is doubtful if these measures would ever be universally accepted.

Another related problem is that of controlling the fertility of persons with severe mental retardation. It has often been suggested that in our society a slow decline in general intelligence is to be expected since those with low intelligence tend to have large families whereas those with high intelligence have small families. However there are valid reasons for rejecting this idea. In the Western hemisphere parents with the largest families are not those with least intelligence but those with about average or even above-average intelligence. Also there is a tendency nowadays for the more highly intelligent to have larger families whereas the severely mentally retarded are usually subfertile or even infertile. A second point is that in multifactorial characters, such as intelligence, the variation in each generation is contributed mainly from the middle of the range. There is no reason to belive that our natural intelligence is declining and no reason for sterilizing the severely mentally retarded because they are usually subfertile anyway.

Finally, there is the question of producing outstanding people by selective breeding or so-called positive eugenics. One way of doing this might be to give tax relief and family allowances to persons with those attributes which we wish to propagate. But here we are faced with the problem of deciding which genes are the ones we wish to increase by selection. There is no guarantee that we will still consider the qualities preferred today important in future generations. Also there is the much more serious problem of how we are going to control such selective breeding programmes. These are complex problems which might well occupy the whole of a book this size. We will therefore limit our discussion to those problems which face the medical geneticist. These include defining and helping to limit the dangers of irradiation and other mutagenic agents and detecting carriers of genetic diseases and persons predisposed to such diseases. These problems will be dealt with in the following chapters.

FURTHER READING

Allison, A. C. (1961). Abnormal haemoglobin and erythrocyte enzyme-deficiency traits. In *Genetical Variation in Human Populations*. Ed. Harrison, G. A., pp. 16–40. London: Pergamon.

Barnicot, N. A. (1961). Haptoglobins and transferrins. In *Genetical Variation in Human Populations*. Ed. Harrison, G. A., pp. 41–61. London: Pergamon.

Candela, P. B. (1942). The introduction of blood group B into Europe. *Hum. Biol.* **14,** 413–443.

Ciba Symposium (1963). *Man and his Future*. Ed. Wolstenholme, G. London: Churchill.

Clarke, B. (1969). The evidence for apostatic selection. *Heredity*, **24,** 347–352.

Clarke, B. (1970). Darwinian evolution of proteins. *Science, N.Y.* **168,** 1009–1011.

Damon, A. (1969). Race, ethnic group and disease. *Social Biol.* **16,** 69–80.

Falconer, D. S. (1960). *Introduction to Quantitative Genetics.* Edinburgh: Oliver and Boyd.

Fisher, R. A. (1958). *The Genetical Theory of Natural Selection.* 2nd ed. New York: Dover.

Ford, E. B. (1960). *Mendelism and Evolution.* London: Methuen.

Gilles, H. M., Fletcher, K. A., Hendrickse, R. G., Linder, R., Reddy, S. and Allan, N. (1967). Glucose-6-phosphate dehydrogenase deficiency, sickling, and malaria in African children in South Western Nigeria. *Lancet*, **1,** 138–140.

Glass, B. (1954). Genetic changes in human populations, especially those due to gene flow and genetic drift. *Adv. Genet.* **6,** 95–139.

Goldschmidt, E. (ed.) (1963). *The Genetics of Migrant and Isolate Populations.* Baltimore: Williams and Wilkins.

Goodman, R. M. (1975). Genetic disorders among the Jewish people. In *Modern Trends in Human Genetics.* Vol. 2. Ed. Emery, A. E. H. pp. 270–307. London: Butterworths.

Haldane, J. B. S. (1961). Natural selection in man. *Prog. med. Genet.* **1,** 27–37.

Harris, H (1969). Enzyme and protein polymorphism in human populations. *Br. med. Bull.* **25**(1), 5–13.

Harris, H. and Kalmus, H. (1951). The distribution of taste thresholds of phenylthio-urea of 384 sib-pairs. *Ann. Eugen.* **16,** 226–230.

Kalmus, H. (1965). *Diagnosis and Genetics of Defective Colour Vision.* London: Pergamon.

Kettlewell, H. B. D. (1965). Insect survival and selection for pattern. *Science, N.Y.* **148,** 1290–1296.

Klein, T. W. and De Frïes, J. C. (1970). Similar polymorphism of taste sensitivity to PTC in mice and men. *Nature, Lond.* **225,** 555–557.

Li, C. C. (1955). *Population Genetics.* Chicago: University of Chicago Press.

Luzzatto, L., Nwachuku-Jarrett, E. S. and Reddy, S. (1970). Increased sickling of parasitised erythrocytes as mechanism of resistance against malaria in the sickle-cell trait. *Lancet*, **1,** 319–321.

McKusick, V. A., Hostetler, J. A., Egeland, J. A. *et al.* (1964). The distribution of certain genes in the Old Order Amish. *Cold Spring Harb. Symp. quant. Biol.* **29,** 99–114.

Mørch, E. T. (1941). *Chondrodystrophic Dwarfs in Denmark.* Copenhagen: Munksgaard.

Neel, J. V. and Post, R. H. (1963). Transitory 'positive' selection for color blindness. *Eugen. Q.* **10**, 33–35.

Norio, R., Nevanlinna, H. R. and Perheentupa, J. (1973). Hereditary diseases in Finland. *Ann. Clin. Res.* **5**, 109–141.

Parsons, P. A. (1964). Genetic regulatory mechanisms at the population level in man. *Science, N.Y.* **146**, 924–925.

Penrose, L. S. (1949). The meaning of 'fitness' in human populations. *Ann. Eugen.* **14**, 301–304.

Penrose, L. S. (1950). Propagation of the unfit. *Lancet*, **2**, 425–427.

Penrose, L. S. (1959). Natural selection in man: some basic problems. In *Natural Selection in Human Populations*. Ed. Roberts, D. F. and Harrison, G. A., pp. 1–10. London: Pergamon.

Reed, T. E. (1969). Caucasian genes in American Negroes. *Science, N.Y.* **165**, 762–768.

Richmond, R. C. (1970). Non-Darwinian evolution: a critique. *Nature, Lond.* **225**, 1025–1028.

Roberts, D. F. (1955). The dynamics of racial intermixture in the American Negro—some anthropological considerations. *Am. J. hum. Genet.* **7**, 361–367.

Roberts, D. F. (1975). Genetic studies of isolates. In *Modern Trends in Human Genetics*. Vol. 2. Ed. Emery, A. E. H. pp. 221-269. London: Butterworths.

Sheppard, P. M. (1967). *Natural Selection and Heredity*. London: Hutchinson.

Vogel, F. (1972). Editor. *Spontaneous Mutation*. New York & Berlin: Springer-Verlag.

Woolf, C. M. and Dukepoo, F. C. (1969). Hopi Indians, inbreeding and albinism. *Science, N.Y.* **164**, 30–37.

X

Radiation and Human Heredity

Since 1945 when the atomic bomb was dropped on Hiroshima and Nagasaki there has been worldwide concern about the hazards of atomic radiation. Before discussing the nature of these hazards let us first be clear about what we mean by ' radiation '.

When we use the word radiation we are usually referring to ' ionizing ' radiations since it is ionizing radiations which cause serious damage to living tissues. Ionizing radiations are so called because they cause each atom they hit to lose an electron, the atom thereby being converted to a positively charged ion. The freed electron is incorporated in another atom which therefore becomes a negatively charged ion. Since each electron lost from one atom is gained by another atom, the number of positively charged ions is equal to the number of negatively charged ions.

Ionizing radiations include electromagnetic waves of very short wavelength (X-rays and gamma rays), and high energy particles (alpha particles, beta particles, and neutrons). X-rays, gamma rays, and neutrons have great penetrating power but alpha particles can penetrate soft tissues to a depth of only a fraction of a millimetre and beta particles only up to a few millimetres in such tissues. However, this does not mean that alpha and beta particles are of no consequence from the point of view of radiation hazards. They are extremely important if they are emitted from a radioactive substance which is actually inside the body.

The amount of radiation received by irradiated tissues is often referred to as the ' dose ' of radiation, which is measured in terms of *rads* and *rems*. The rad is a measure of the amount of any ionizing radiation which is actually *absorbed* by the tissues. One rad is equivalent to 100 ergs of energy absorbed per gram of tissue. Many biological effects of ionizing radiations depend on the volume of tissue exposed. In man irradiation of the whole body with a dose of 300–500 rads is usually fatal, but in the treatment of malignant tumours as much as 10,000 rads may be given to a *small* volume of tissue without serious effects.

Man is liable to be exposed to a mixture of radiations and the rem is a convenient unit for it is a measure of *any* radiation in terms of X-rays. A rem of radiation is that absorbed dose which produces in a given tissue the same biological effect as one rad of X-rays. Expressing doses of radiation in terms of rems permits us to compare the amounts of different types of radiation to which man is exposed. A millirem (mrem) is one-thousandth of a rem.

SOURCES OF IONIZING RADIATIONS

It is useful to consider sources of ionizing radiations as falling into two classes: natural (background) and artificial. There is every reason to believe that the amount of radiation from natural sources has remained the same since life first appeared on this planet. These natural sources of radiation include cosmic rays, external radiation from radioactive materials in certain rocks, and internal radiation from radioactive materials in our tissues. The amount of radiation from these sources absorbed by different organs of the body is about the same.

Cosmic rays originate from outer space and have such great penetrating powers that the amount received by the body is practically the same outdoors as it is indoors. These rays have been detected in mines over a quarter of a mile deep. As would be expected, the intensity of these rays increases with altitude and at 10,000 feet the intensity is about three times that at sea level. At present the effects of cosmic radiation in man are probably negligible but in the future the hazards to aircrews who operate at very high altitudes for considerable periods of time may be significant. The effects on persons involved in interplanetary space travel will have to be carefully studied. The intensity of cosmic radiation depends not only on altitude but also on latitude being greater at the poles than at the equator. It is therefore difficult to give an average figure but very roughly the dose to the gonads is about 30 mrem per year from cosmic radiation. The dose of radiation is expressed in relation to the amount received by the gonads because, as we shall see later, it is the *genetic* effects of radiation which are so important. The gonad dose of radiation is often expressed as the amount received in 30 years. This period of time has been chosen because it corresponds roughly to the generation time in man. In the case of cosmic radiation the dose to the gonads is about 0·90 rems per 30 years.

Various natural radioactive elements such as thorium, uranium, radium, and an isotope of potassium (K^{40}) are widely distributed over the earth's surface. The amount of radiation received by man from these sources varies considerably in different parts of the world depending on the amounts of these radioactive substances in different rocks and soils. For example the amount of radiation from granite is considerably more than from limestone. An average dose to the gonads from radiation from naturally occurring radioactive materials external to the body amounts to about 50 mrems per year or 1·50 rems in 30 years. However, very much higher levels are to be found in certain regions of the world where there are comparatively large amounts of radioactive substances in the soil and rock formations. For example in the state of Espírito Santo in Brazil the average level of radiation is about 500 mrems per year and in parts of the state of Kerala in southwest India it is as high as 2800 mrems per year.

Certain natural radioactive materials are constituents of the air we breath, the food we eat, and the water we drink. These radioactive materials include minute quantities of uranium, thorium and related substances, and isotopes of potassium (K^{40}), strontium (Sr^{90}), and carbon (C^{14}). Altogether the radiation from these elements within the body amounts to about 20 mrems per year or 0·60 rems in 30 years. It has been estimated that the average total dose of radiation received by the gonads from all natural sources, whether external to the body or internal, amounts to about 100 mrems per year or 3 rems in 30 years.

Turning now to artificial or man-made sources of radiation these include medical radiology, occupational exposure, and fallout from nuclear explosions. The hazards and dangers from radioactive fallout resulting from the testing of nuclear weapons has become a major political issue in many countries, but the intention in this discussion is to present some of the relevant scientific facts rather than to discuss the moral and other implications of weapon testing. As we shall see later, on the average the world population at present is exposed to less radiation from fallout from nuclear explosions than from medical radiology. This does not mean that radioactive fallout is of no importance, but it does mean that dangers from this source should be considered in perspective so that other sources of danger are not overshadowed and possibly ignored.

When a nuclear device is detonated, it releases a tremendous amount of energy in the form of heat, light, ionizing radiations, and many radioactive substances. Among the most important of these radioactive substances are isotopes of carbon (C^{14}), iodine (I^{131}), cesium (Cs^{137}), and strontium (Sr^{90}). Cs^{137} and Sr^{90} are considered most important because they are liberated in very large amounts and remain radioactive for many years. The 'half-life' of Sr^{90} for example is 28 years and that of Cs^{137} is 30 years. This means that the radioactivity of Sr^{90} is reduced by a half in 28 years, by three-quarters in 56 years and by seven-eighths in 84 years. The hot gases of a nuclear explosion carry these radioactive substances into the atmosphere and stratosphere where they remain for some time before falling back to the earth (fallout). Due to air-currents radioactive fallout is not limited to the immediate locality of the nuclear explosion but is ultimately worldwide. Cs^{137} and Sr^{90} are deposited on water which is later drunk or on vegetation which is either eaten by man or by cattle. The radioactive materials may also be passed on to man in the meat of cattle or in their milk. In man Cs^{137} is widely distributed throughout the body but is particularly abundant in muscle whereas Sr^{90} becomes almost entirely localized in bone. It is difficult to determine the precise amount of radiation to the gonads from nuclear fallout but one authority estimates that the fallout from a high yield atmospheric test explosion is roughly 3·0 mrem or 3 per cent of one year's unavoidable exposure to natural background. At the present moment the gonad dose of radiation from radioactive fallout is considerably less than from any of the sources of background radiation (table XIX).

Table XIX. *Approximate average doses of ionizing radiation from various sources to the gonads of the general population*

Source of radiation	Average dose per year (mrems)	Average dose per 30 years (rems)
Natural:		
Cosmic radiation	30	0·90
External gamma radiation	50	1·50
Internal gamma radiation	20	0·60
Artificial:		
Medical radiology	35	1·05
Radioactive fallout	1	0·03
Occupational and miscellaneous	2	0·06
Total	138	4·14

Of particular importance, both in magnitude and since control is considerably easier, is the radiation dose to the population from medical radiology. Radiography is an essential diagnostic tool in medical practice and its potential hazards have to be carefully weighed against the great amount of obvious good which results from such investigations. It is very much easier to obtain a figure for the radiation dose to the patient resulting from a particular type of X-ray examination than it is to give an estimate of the reduction in suffering which results from the use of such a test. Nevertheless this is not to underestimate the potential hazards of radiography although the medical profession in many countries takes great care to minimize exposure to X-rays during radiographic examinations. In particular the dose to the gonads is very carefully controlled. The problem in the case of radiotherapy is a little different. Here various forms of external irradiation and internal irradiation from the administration of radioactive substances such as iodine-131, phosphorous-32 and gold-198 are used mainly for the treatment of malignant tumours. Since patients who undergo such treatment are usually past the child-bearing age the genetic hazards of radiation are not so important.

The average population dose to the gonads from medical radiology (both diagnostic and therapeutic) has been estimated to be about 35 mrems per year or 1·05 rems in 30 years. These are *average* figures for highly developed countries. Some individuals receive no radiation at all from this source throughout their entire lives whereas others may accumulate a considerable dose. The average gonad dose from medical radiology in some countries (U.S.A.) is greater than in other countries (U.K.).

Finally another source of harmful radiation is to be found in certain occupations. Considerable numbers of workers are engaged in medical radiology and atomic energy projects. The use of X-rays for detecting flaws in castings and for the examination of other commercial products has introduced potential hazards in industry. The use of radioactive isotopes has increased greatly in many spheres of activity from biologists using tritiated thymidine in studies of chromosome replication to engineers interested in the combustion of motor fuels. Even persons not exposed to radiation in their everyday occupation may receive very small amounts from luminous dials on wrist watches and from television screens. The average population dose to the gonads from occupational exposure and miscellaneous sources is about 2·0 mrems per year or 0·06 rems in 30 years. Obviously persons in technologically advanced countries will be exposed to the greatest amount of radiation from man-made sources.

EFFECTS OF RADIATION

Ionizing radiations affect both the cells of the body and the sex cells; they have somatic and genetic effects. The immediate somatic effects of acute *whole* body irradiation were seen in those individuals close to the centre of the atomic explosions in Japan in 1945. Of those who were not killed immediately by the blast, many suffered from the effects of having received an enormous dose of radiation. Some died within 10 days, others were ill for several weeks. Those exposed lost their hair and their bone marrow activity was greatly reduced so that the number of circulating leucocytes was considerably diminished and their resistance to infection was therefore severely impaired. Among those who recovered from the immediate effects some later developed leukaemia. One of the possible dangers of radiotherapy is an increased risk of developing leukaemia or other neoplastic diseases. Experiments on animals have shown that exposure to ionizing radiation leads to a reduction in the life span but so far there is no evidence of this in man. There is good evidence in man that irradiation of the fetus, particularly during the early weeks of pregnancy, is associated with an increased risk of microcephaly (p. 202) and malignant disease in childhood. For this reason it is recommended that X-ray examination of the lower abdomen should be carried out within 10 days following the first day of the last menstrual period when it is most improbable that the woman could be pregnant.

The somatic effects of a high dose of radiation to a *localized* volume of tissue are seen in patients being treated for malignant tumours and in persons involved in accidents with radioactive materials. The result may be local tissue necrosis (radiation burn) and general malaise with some nausea and vomiting (radiation sickness). In the treatment of malignant tumours the somatic effects of irradiation are kept to a minimum by carefully controlling the dose to any given area of skin and by giving drugs which reduce the symptoms of radiation sickness. Sufficient exposure to radiation will cause sterility but since it requires several hundred rads to destroy the sex cells, if this amount of radiation were received by the whole body it would probably be fatal. Radiotherapists take great care to avoid all unnecessary irradiation of the gonads when giving local treatment.

The somatic effects of radiation are extremely important to those involved in radiotherapy and the handling of radioactive materials but our main concern here is with the genetic effects.

In 1927 H. J. Muller demonstrated that exposure of colonies of *Drosophila* to X-rays resulted in an increase in the number of mutations in excess of those occurring spontaneously. He thus showed that X-rays are mutagenic and for his work in the field of radiation genetics he was awarded the Nobel prize in 1946.

For convenience a mutation was defined earlier as a change in a gene, but this is only partly true. Mutations are of two kinds— chromosome aberrations and point mutations. The former are gross structural changes of the chromosomes such as deletions and breakages which are caused by high doses of radiation. They may be found in the blood of patients who have undergone radiotherapy. However, when we speak about mutations in the present context we usually mean point mutations: a change which involves a single gene locus or at the most a minute region of the chromosome involving a few adjacent loci. Point mutations involve such a minute amount of chromosome material that they produce no visible change microscopically. It seems that ionizing radiations and other mutagenic agents (exposure to high temperatures, ultraviolet radiation, and certain chemicals have been shown to be mutagenic in animals) bring about their effects by changing the arrangement of the atoms within a localized region of the DNA molecule. Mutations are usually harmful. Perhaps because evolutionary processes have resulted in a genetic make-up which is best adapted to the environment in which the organism lives, any upset of such a balance would be detrimental. But not all mutations are detrimental.

Sometimes a new mutation is beneficial. Plant and animal breeders are continually on the lookout for new mutations which may be of economic importance. Examples include strains of wheat which are resistant to black stem rust disease, or have increased yield and improved baking qualities; strains of flax with long fibres; strains of barley with higher protein content; varieties of cattle with increased milk yield. There is no doubt that these mutations are beneficial to *man*, but it is a moot point whether, under natural conditions, such mutations are necessarily of benefit to the organism possessing them. In man a new mutation is much more likely to be recognized if its effect is detrimental rather than if it confers some increased resistance to infection or leads to a slightly longer survival time.

Experiments with animals and plants have shown that the number of mutations produced by irradiation is proportional to the dose; the larger the dose the more mutations are produced. One important point is that there is *no* threshold below which irradiation has no effect. It is believed that even the smallest dose of radiation may produce a mutation. The effect of ionizing radiations can be likened to firing a rifle at random at objects in a shooting gallery. The more shots we fire the more likely we are to hit something (cause a mutation). If we were to fire only a single shot there is still a possibility that we might hit something but this is far less than if we were able to fire many shots. In the latter case we are not only more likely to hit one object but we are also more likely to hit several objects. When a person has a chest X-ray most of the radiation passes straight through his chest, but because some of the rays are deflected and scattered, a small amount of radiation may reach the gonads. This small amount of radiation will not necessarily cause a mutation but there is a small possibility that it might, and if a *large* section of the community have chest X-rays it is quite possible that a few new mutations will result. The genetic effects of ionizing radiations are cumulative so that each time a person is exposed to radiation the dose he receives has to be added to the amount of radiation he has already received. The total number of radiation-induced mutations is directly proportional to the *total* gonad dosage.

In all living organisms which have been investigated, from bacteriophage to man, mutations occur very rarely under natural conditions. These naturally occurring mutations are referred to as *spontaneous* mutations. Obviously there must be a cause for such mutations and it would seem reasonable to implicate background radiation. However, as we shall see later, natural background levels of radiation are probably too low to account for the vast majority of spontaneously occurring mutations.

Experiments on *Drosophila* have shown that ionizing radiations may cause mutations not only in the sex cells but also in the body cells. Mutations induced in the body cells (*somatic mutations*) are confined to these cells and are not transferred to the sex cells and therefore not transmitted to future progeny. There appears to be no authenticated case of radiation-induced somatic mutation in man, unless we consider leukaemia the result of a somatic mutation in the blood-forming cells.

ASSESSMENT OF THE GENETIC EFFECTS OF RADIATION IN MAN

In an attempt to relate the potential genetic hazards of exposure quantitatively to ionizing radiations scientists have introduced the concepts of *gonad* dose, *genetic* dose, and *doubling* dose. The gonad dose is that dose of radiation received by the gonads when a person is subjected to a particular radiological examination. It is determined by placing instruments for measuring the amount of radiation at appropriate sites on the body. A model of a human body made of plastic, or some such material, is often used to assess the dose to the ovaries. The gonad dose depends of course on the type of examination. For example the gonad dose from a kidney X-ray is many times greater than the dose from a chest X-ray. From the genetic point of view we have seen that the gonad dose is often expressed in terms of the amount of radiation received by the gonads over a period of 30 years.

Whereas gonad dose refers to the radiation received by the individual, the genetic dose refers to the gonad dose spread over the whole population. The genetic dose can be calculated from appropriate formulae, For example in the case of diagnostic radiology, in order to calculate the genetic dose we have to know the number of persons examined radiologically per year according to sex, age, and type of examination, the expected number of children still to be born to an average person of the same age and sex, the average dose received by the gonads per examination and the number of persons of the same age and sex in the general population. Estimates of the gonad dose and genetic dose for particular procedures have permitted comparisons to be made of the possible genetic hazards of various radiological procedures.

In estimating the genetic hazards of ionizing radiation in man there has been the difficulty of extrapolating data from mutation rates obtained in lower organisms which vary considerably. However, the radiation induced mutation rates for bacteria, fungi, *Drosophila*, higher plants and mammals are essentially the same if expressed in terms of the amount of DNA per nucleus (fig. 45)

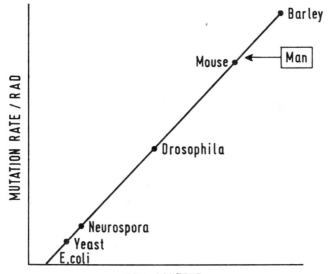

Figure 45. Mutation rates for various organisms expressed in terms of the amount of DNA per nucleus. (Data from S. Abrahamson and published with permission.)

and knowing the amount of DNA per nucleus in man (2·9 pg per haploid genome) it is possible to estimate the mutation rate per locus per rad (i.e. $2·6 \times 10^{-7}$) (Abrahamson *et al.*, 1973).

The *doubling dose* is the amount of radiation which would be expected to double the present spontaneous mutation rate. There is nothing especially significant about 'doubling' the mutation rate. We could quite easily have chosen some other multiple. However, the doubling dose is usually chosen as an arbitrary standard. In the mouse, but not in *Drosophila*, the mutagenic

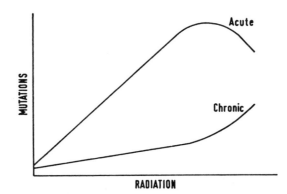

Figure 46. The effects of acute and chronic exposure to radiation on the production of mutations in animals.

effect of a given dose of ionizing radiation depends on whether the dose is given in a very brief period of time or is given at a lower intensity but over a long period of time. The former is referred to as acute radiation, the latter as chronic radiation. In the mouse an acute dose of high-intensity radiation produces about four times as many mutations as the same dose applied chronically at low intensity (fig. 46). Based on the data obtained from these experiments it has been estimated that the chronic doubling dose in man is probably about 100 rems. Now we have seen already that man receives only about 3 rems of radiation from background sources over a 30-year period. This amount of radiation would therefore account for only 3 per cent of the spontaneous mutation rate. *The majority of spontaneous mutations in man must therefore be due to causes other than background radiation.*

In man *chemical mutagenesis* may in fact be more important than radiation induced genetic damage. Experiments have shown that certain chemicals such as mustard gas, formaldehyde, some basic

dyes and even caffeine are mutagenic in animals, and many mutagenic substances are present in various agricultural, industrial and
pharmaceutical chemicals in use today. Perhaps certain metabolites
produced within the body affect the nuclei of the germ cells and thus
cause mutation. However, in man nothing is known of the effects
of chemicals on the induction of mutations but consideration of
animal data makes this seem very likely.

High temperature is known to increase the mutation rate in
animals but again the relevance of this to man is conjectural. It
has been found in man that scrotal skin temperatures are significantly
higher in those who wear trousers than in those who wear kilts and
therefore perhaps the mutation rates are different in the two groups.
However this is all in the realm of speculation and at the present
moment we are unable to account for the vast majority of mutations
in man.

The genetic effects of radiation are not easy to assess for they are
not manifest in the generation which is exposed to radiation but
in subsequent generations. If a dominant mutation is produced then
it will be manifest in the next generation but a recessive mutation
is only likely to be manifest when two heterozygotes marry and
have children. If the recessive mutant gene is very rare then the
chance of this happening will be small. Each one of us carries
recessive mutant genes which in the homozygous state would have
very serious effects. Experiments with *Drosophila* have shown that
natural populations of this organism carry a large number of harmful
mutant genes which are concealed in the heterozygous state. Some
authorities have estimated that in man each individual carries about
six lethal or semilethal genes. These estimates are very conservative
and the actual figure may be many times greater. Harmful genes of
all kinds constitute the so-called *genetic load* of the population.
When we consider the genetic effects of radiation we have to determine to what extent this factor influences the genetic load of the
population.

Neel and Schull tackled the problem by comparing the offspring
of parents exposed to atomic radiation at the time Hiroshima and
Nagasaki were bombed with those of parents who were not exposed
to radiation. Analysis of several thousands of births revealed no
significant differences in the incidence of stillbirths, congenital malformations, or neonatal deaths. This does not mean, however, that
there are no genetic consequences of atomic radiation. A number
of autosomal recessive mutants may have been produced but they
will not be manifest for several generations. However, recessive
mutations produced on the X chromosome would be immediately

manifest in hemizygous male offspring of mothers who had been irradiated. If these mutants were lethal then the number of male births would be diminished; the sex ratio (number of male births divided by the number of female births) would be reduced. This is what would be expected if recessive X-linked mutations were produced in the maternal gonad of a woman who had been irradiated. If X-linked dominant lethal mutations were produced then there would be an equal chance of both male and female babies being eliminated and the sex ratio would remain unchanged. Recessive X-linked lethal genes in the *paternal* gonads would have no effect on the sex ratio but dominant X-linked lethal mutations would lead to an excess of live male births with a resultant increase in the sex ratio. In other words if a large enough sample were studied one would expect that in the case of fathers exposed to radiation the sex ratio of their offspring would be increased, whereas in the case of mothers exposed to radiation the sex ratio of their offspring would be decreased.

In the study of parents who had been exposed to atomic radiation in Japan, evidence was obtained by Neel and Schull of slight changes in the sex ratio which could be interpreted as being due to the production of X-linked mutations. In non-irradiated parents the sex ratio of their offspring was 0·5209 but in those parents who had received a dose of about 200 rads the sex ratio of their offspring was 0·5272 when the father had been irradiated and 0·5119 when the mother had been irradiated.

However, in an extended study published in 1966, these investigators were unable to confirm the effect of radiation on the sex ratio.

In France a study has been made of the sex ratio in offspring of parents who have had radiotherapy of the pelvis for various reasons. The results were similar to those obtained in the earlier Japanese study: there was a slight increase in the sex ratio when the father was the irradiated parent and a slight decrease when the mother was the irradiated parent. However the results of such studies have to be accepted with caution because many factors other than radiation may influence the sex ratio. For instance the sex ratio is influenced by paternal (but not maternal) age. It is also related to birth order, the proportion of males being highest in first births and decreasing with successive births. In studies of the sex ratio there is always the difficulty of choosing appropriately matched controls.

Other attempts to detect genetic damage resulting from radiation have been made in the United States by comparing the incidence of abortions, stillbirths, and congenital malformations in the offspring of radiologists and in the offspring of other medical specialists. The assumption made was that radiologists are exposed to more radiation than are other physicians. The results of these studies showed that there were slightly more fetal deaths (abortions and stillbirths) and congenital malformations in the offspring of radiologists but the differences were not statistically significant. Recent claims that Sr^{90} fallout from nuclear tests may have had a significant effect on infant mortality in the United States since 1945 has not stood up to critical evaluation. Recent animal studies have also failed to demonstrate any significant genetic effects of the increased amounts of background radiation in Kerala in southwest India.

Thus we can see that so far attempts to demonstrate that radiation causes genetic damage in man have not been very convincing though there is some evidence that exposure to X-irradiation may predispose to non-disjunction in man (see p. 64). This does not mean however that radiation does not cause genetic damage in man. As we have seen already experiments on other organisms have shown quite clearly that ionizing radiations do cause mutations, the vast majority of which are harmful. The important point as far as man is concerned is that induced mutations may harm individuals in future generations. The hazard is not so much to ourselves as to descendants. Unfortunately, in man we do not have any *precise* way of estimating the amount of genetic damage caused by radiation.

The International Commission of Radiological Protection (ICRP) working in close liaison with various agencies of the United Nations (WHO, UNESCO, IAEA, etc.) has been mainly responsible for defining what is referred to as the *maximum permissible dose* of radiation. The maximum permissible genetic dose of radiation is an arbitrary safety limit and is probably very much less than that which would cause any significant effect on the frequency of harmful mutations within the population. It has been recommended that the genetic dose to the whole population from all sources, additional to natural background radiation, should not exceed 5 rems over a period of 30 years.

There is no doubting the potential dangers, both somatic and genetic, of excessive exposure to ionizing radiations. In the case of medical radiology the dose of radiation resulting from a particular procedure has to be weighed against the ultimate beneficial effects to the patient. In the case of occupational exposure to radiation, the answer lies in defining the risks and introducing adequate legislation. With regard to the dangers from fallout from nuclear explosions the solution would seem obvious.

FURTHER READING

Abrahamson, S., *et al.* (1973). Uniformity of radiation-induced mutation rates among different species. *Nature* **245**, 460-462.

Alexander, P. (1965). *Atomic Radiation and Life.* 2nd ed. London: Penguin Books.

Court Brown, W. M., *et al.* (1965). Quantitative studies of chromosome aberrations in man following acute and chronic exposure to x-rays and gamma rays. *Lancet*, **1**, 1239–1241.

Crow, J. F. (1955). A comparison of fetal and infant death rates in the progeny of radiologists and pathologists. *Am. J. Roentg.* **73**, 467–471.

Crow, J. F. (1961). Mutation in man. *Prog. med. Genet.* **1**, 1–26.

Dye, D. L. and Wilkinson, M. (1965). Radiation hazards in space. *Science, N.Y.* **147**, 19–25.

Grüneberg, H. *et al.* (1966). *A Search for Genetic Effects of High Natural Radioactivity in South India.* London: Her Majesty's Stationery Office.

James, A. P. and Newcombe, H. B. (1964). The quantitative assessment of hereditary damage induced by radiation. *Prog. med. Genet.* **3**, 217–259.

Kato, H., Schull, W. J. and Neel, J. V. (1966). A cohort-type study of survival in the children of parents exposed to atomic bombings. *Am. J. hum. Genet.* **18**, 339–373.

Lindop, P. J. and Rotblat, J. (1969). Strontium-90 and infant mortality. *Nature, London.* **224**, 1257–1260.

Loutit, J. F. (1962). *Irradiation of Mice and Men.* Chicago: University of Chicago Press.

Macht, S. H. and Lawrence, P. S. (1955). National survey of congenital malformations resulting from exposure to roentgen radiation. *Am. J. Roentg.* **73**, 442–466.

Mayneord, W. V. (1964). *Radiation and Health.* London: Nuffield Provincial Hospitals Trust.

Medical Research Council (1960). *The Hazards to Man of Nuclear and Allied Radiations.* London: Her Majesty's Stationery Office.

Penrose, L. S. (1961). Mutation. In *Recent Advances in Human Genetics.* Ed. Penrose, L. S., pp. 1–18. London: Churchill.

Purdom, C. E. (1963). *Genetic Effects of Radiations.* London: Newnes.

Schull, W. J., Neel, J. V. and Hashizume, A. (1966). Some further observations on the sex-ratio among infants born to survivors of the atomic bombings of Hiroshima and Nagasaki. *Am. J. hum. Genet.* **18**, 328–338.

Spar, I. L. (1969). Genetic effects of radiation. *Med. Clins N. Am.* **53**(4), 956–976.

Stevenson, A. C. (1958). The genetic hazards of radiation. *Practitioner,* **181**, 559–571.

Turpin, R., Lejeune, J. and Rethore, M. O. (1956). Étude de la descendance de sujets traitéts par radiotherapie pelvienne. *Acta genet. Statist. med.* **6**, 204–216.

United Nations (1962). *Report of the Scientific Committee on the Effects of Atomic Radiation.* New York.

World Health Organization (1962). *Radiation Hazards in Perspective.* Technical report series No. 248. Geneva.

XI

Genetics and the Physician

Because of advances in medicine and surgery, diseases due to infections and nutritional deficiencies are gradually being controlled. Environmental diseases are being displaced by others which are largely or even entirely genetically determined (Roberts *et al.*, 1970).

The extent of the problem can be judged from the data in table XX. Roughly 1 in 20 children admitted to hospital has a disorder which is entirely genetic in origin and such disorders account for about 1 in 10 of childhood deaths in hospital. However, only about 1 in 100 adult inpatients has a unifactorial or chromosome disorder, but then many of these disorders lead to early death or if they are compatible with survival to adulthood they usually do not warrant hospital admission. Most genetic disorders affecting adults have a multifactorial basis.

There has been a change in the sort of problems the physician encounters in his practice. Congenital abnormalities and hereditary disorders are becoming of increasing importance and the physician is being asked more and more often to give advice concerning genetic problems. Such problems may involve the advisability of cousin marriages, delayed or abnormal sexual development, recurrent abortion, child adoption, paternity determination, and particularly the risks of recurrence in certain hereditary diseases. There are now many centres throughout the world with genetic counselling clinics which deal specifically with these problems. In this chapter we shall see how our knowledge of genetics is applied to answering some of these problems.

Genetic Counselling

The genetic counsellor faced with a couple who need advice is concerned with three problems. Firstly, he establishes a precise diagnosis based on the results of clinical examination and relevant laboratory investigations. Secondly, he discusses the prognosis and availability and value of any possible treatments. Finally, he determines the risks of recurrence, explains the genetic implications, relieves feelings of guilt and with understanding and sympathy helps

Table XX. *Incidence of genetic disorders among various groups of patients*
(UF=unifactorial; CHR=chromosomal; MF=multifactorial)

Region	Year	Patients surveyed	Total No. of patients	Proportion (%) of cases		
				UF	CHR	MF
Montreal	1970	Paediatric in-patients	1145	6·7	0·4	3·9
Los Angeles	1971-2	Paediatric in-patients	1500	3·0	0·5	15·0
Boston	1970	Paediatric in-patients	200	5·0	0·0	16·5
		Paediatric out-patients	200	2·5	0·0	14·5
		Adult in-patients	200	1·5	0·0	—
		Adult out-patients	200	1·0	0·5	—
London	1954	Childhood deaths in hospital	200	12·0		25·5
Newcastle	1960-6	Childhood deaths in hospital	1041	8·5	2·5	31.0
Edinburgh	1971	Adult in-patients*	7126	0·3	0·2	11·9

* Excludes obstetrics, gynaecology and psychiatry.

the parents to arrive at a decision. Thus the determination of the risks of recurrence, though important, is only one aspect of counselling. The decision whether or not to accept the risks is usually left to the parents.

CALCULATING PROBABILITIES

From the point of view of calculating the risks of recurrence, or the *probability* of being affected which is the same thing, hereditary diseases can be divided into two groups. In the first group the mode of inheritance is simple (autosomal dominant, autosomal recessive, or X-linked) and the risks of recurrence are easily calculated but most of these diseases are rare. In the second group there is no doubt that heredity plays an important part in aetiology but they are not inherited in any simple manner and the recurrence risks are derived from observations on the frequency of the disease in relatives of affected persons (empiric risks). This latter group includes many common diseases. The risks of recurrence in the first group are high, whereas they are usually low in the second group. Fortunately the risks of recurrence are usually small in those conditions in which the risks are most difficult to estimate.

In those conditions inherited in a simple manner it is important to remember that chance has no memory. For example, if a father and mother are both heterozygous for the same recessive gene the chance of their having an affected child is 1 in 4 with each pregnancy. This is true irrespective of whether or not they have already had any affected children.

When we discuss the probability of a person's being affected we usually mean the *prior* probability; that is, the probability based on our knowledge of the person's antecedents. For the sake of simplicity this custom will be adopted in later discussions. However, it should be noted that more precise estimates of the chances of recurrence can be made by also taking into account the so-called conditional probability; that is, the probability that persons may be affected (or be carriers) depending on their age, or the results of various biochemical tests or whether or not any of their children have been affected. From our knowledge of the prior and conditional probabilities it is possible to calculate the *joint* probability, which is the product of the prior and conditional probabilities, and finally the *posterior* or *relative* probability which is the joint probability of being affected (or of being a carrier) divided by the joint probability of not being affected plus the joint probability of being affected.

The procedure is illustrated in the following example. A man aged 50, whose father died of Huntington's chorea, wishes to know what the chances are of his own son developing this disease. Huntington's chorea is inherited as an autosomal dominant trait the first signs of which usually appear some time between the ages of 25 and 55. Now the chances of his having inherited the mutant gene from his father (the prior probability) is half. Since approximately 80 per cent of cases of Huntington's chorea develop symptoms before the age of 50 the chance (conditional probability) that he would not have manifested the disease by this age, even if he had inherited the gene is about one-fifth. The joint probability of having inherited the disease and appearing normal is therefore one-tenth. The prior probability of *not* having inherited the disease is half, the conditional probability of being normal if he has *not* inherited the disease is of course 1, and the joint probability is therefore half. The posterior or relative probability of having inherited the disease is one-sixth.

Probability	Inherited the disorder	Not inherited the disorder
Prior	1/2	1/2
Conditional	1/5	1
Joint	1/10	1/2
Relative	$\dfrac{1/10}{1/10+1/2}=1/6$	

The probability that his son will be affected is therefore 1 in 12 or 8·5 per cent. Of course as each year goes by and the father remains healthy so his risks of having inherited Huntington's chorea decrease (fig. 47).

A computer program *PEDIG* (Heuch & Li, 1972) has been developed which can deal with risk calculations of this kind. It can deal with any disorder where the mode of inheritance is simple, and information on age of onset and other characteristics can be included. Such involved calculations however, are not necessary when the disorder is fully penetrant and age of onset does not present a problem.

GENETIC COUNSELLING IN RARE DISEASES

1. *Autosomal Dominant Disorders*
In a person heterozygous for an autosomal dominant gene the probability of any of his children being similarly affected is half. If the parents already have an affected child the probability that any

future child will be affected is also half. Further, assuming that the gene in question is always fully penetrant, then the unaffected child of an affected parent cannot be a heterozygote and therefore cannot transmit the disease to his own children. Unfortunately in some hereditary disorders, the mutant gene may not be fully penetrant in some individuals who may thus appear perfectly healthy even though they carry the gene. A very careful clinical examination is essential in such cases for occasionally a person said by his relatives to be perfectly healthy may in fact be very slightly affected. Such

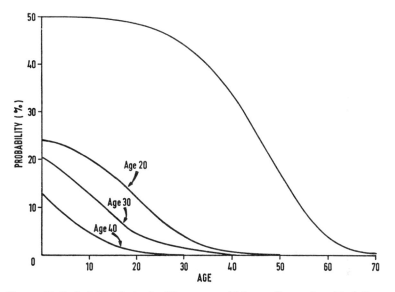

Figure 47. Probability that a healthy man and his son (born when his father was aged, 20, 30 or 40 years) may have inherited Huntington's chorea from a grandparent.

an extremely mild expression of a disease is sometimes referred to as a ' forme fruste '. In some instances even after the most careful and thorough clinical examination no evidence of the disease in question may be found even though the individual is known to carry the gene because, as an example, he may have an affected parent and an affected child. In such cases the gene is truly non-penetrant. Genetic counselling in regard to those diseases which may not always be fully penetrant can be very difficult.

Some autosomal dominant traits are said to exhibit the pheno-menon of *anticipation;* that is, the onset of the disease occurs at an earlier age in the offspring than in the parents. Since early onset is usually associated with increased severity, in certain diseases (such as myotonic dystrophy) it may seem that there is a progressive worsening of the condition with each succeeding generation. However, this is merely due to the way in which cases are collected for study. Thus, only those individuals who are less severely affected tend to have children a proportion of whom will also be affected, some severely so. Secondly, those patients in whom the disease begins earlier and is more severe are more likely to be ascertained. Finally, because the observer and the observed are in the same generation many sibs who at present appear to be unaffected may develop the disease later in life.

2. Autosomal Recessive Disorders

With an autosomal recessive condition the parents of an affected child are both heterozygotes. There is one possible exception and that is when only one of the parents is a heterozygote, and a muta-

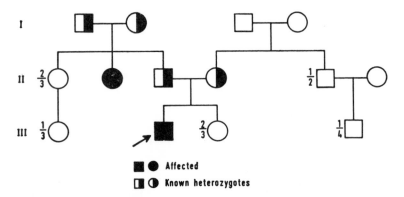

Figure 48. The probabilities of various relatives being carriers of an autosomal recessive trait. For example, an unaffected sib has a 2 in 3 chance of being a carrier. *Note*, since II_4 is a carrier therefore I_3 or I_4 must be a carrier.

tion occurs in the gamete from the other parent but this would be an extremely rare event. In phenylketonuria this would be some 500 times less likely than the marriage of two heterozygotes. When both parents are heterozygotes the chance of their having an affected child is 1 in 4. Since most families nowadays are small, autosomal recessive conditions may often appear as 'sporadic' or isolated cases. It is quite common for only one person to be affected in a family.

The probabilities of various relatives of an affected individual being carriers of an autosomal recessive trait are shown in fig. 48. The probability of having an affected child is the product of the probabilities of the parents being carriers multiplied by $\frac{1}{4}$. Thus the probability of an unaffected sib being a carrier is $\frac{2}{3}$. If the probability of a particular cousin being a carrier is $\frac{1}{4}$ then if the cousins marry each other the risk to each child of being affected is $\frac{2}{3} \times \frac{1}{4} \times \frac{1}{4} = 1$ in 24.

3. X-Linked Disorders

In severe X-linked recessive disorders affected males are either infertile or do not live long enough to marry. In either event these disorders are usually transmitted by healthy female carriers. The carrier of an X-linked disorder transmits the gene to half her daughters who are therefore carriers and to half her sons who will thus be affected. If an affected male does have children his sons are never affected but all his daughters are carriers (fig. 49).

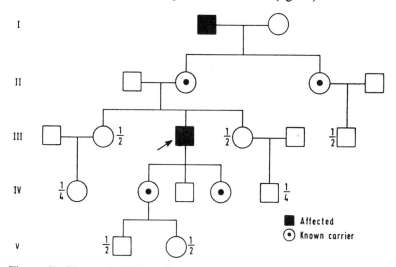

Figure 49. The probabilities of male relatives being affected and female relatives being carriers of an X-linked recessive trait. All the daughters of an affected male are definite carriers.

If a woman has only one affected son this might be the result of a new mutation, in which case, since it is very unlikely that a mutation will recur, any future children might be expected to be perfectly normal. Though there are now tests by means of which it is possible to recognize a proportion of carriers of several X-linked conditions (p. 202), unfortunately none will prove with certainty that a woman is *not* a carrier because of X-inactivation of the X chromosome (see p. 86).

The fact that in many X-linked disorders only a proportion of carriers can be detected by special tests poses a problem if a suspected carrier has a normal test result. This can be resolved in a manner similar to that used in calculating risks in a disorder such as Huntington's chorea where there is a variable age of onset (p. 195). In an X-linked lethal disorder, such as Duchenne muscular dystrophy, the prior probability of a woman being a carrier as the result of a new mutation in either her father's sperm or her mother's ovum is 2μ where μ is the mutation rate and is approximately equal to 5×10^{-5} in the case of Duchenne muscular dystrophy. The probability that she might have inherited the mutant gene from her mother is also 2μ and therefore the total *prior* probability of her being a carrier is 4μ and of not being a carrier is $(1-4\mu)$ which is approximately equal to unity. The conditional probability can be subdivided into genetic and test result probabilities. The genetic probability of her having, for example, one normal and one affected son is $(\frac{1}{2})^2$ if she is a carrier, and equal to the mutation rate if she is not a carrier. The test result probability is calculated from knowing the distribution of test results in controls and known carriers. Thus if her serum level of creatine kinase were 25 units the likelihood of this if she were not a carrier is 0·48 and if she were a carrier is 0·07 since 48 per cent of controls and 7 per cent of carriers have serum creatine kinase levels in this region. The probability of her being a carrier can therefore be calculated as follows:

Probability	Carrier	Not a carrier
Prior	4μ	$1\text{-}4\mu \simeq 1$
Conditional:		
genetic	$\frac{1}{4}$	μ (new mutation)
biochemical	0·07	0·48
Joint	$(0\cdot07)\mu$	$(0\cdot48)\mu$

$$\text{Relative} \quad \frac{(0\cdot07)\mu}{(0\cdot07)\mu + (0\cdot48)\mu} \simeq 0\cdot13 \text{ or 1 in 8}$$

It can be shown that if a woman has an *affected son* but no one else in the family is affected, and if ' h ' is the relative probability of normal homozygosity to heterozygosity for a particular test result (i.e. 48/7 or 6·8 in the above example) and if 'r' is the number of normal sons, then the probability of her being a carrier is

$$\frac{2}{2+h2^r}$$

Methods for calculating risks in various family situations where there is only one affected person in a family have been published (Emery, 1969). The distinction between an autosomal recessive condition and an X-linked condition is important. If the condition is due to an autosomal recessive gene the normal sister of an affected male, even if she is a carrier, is unlikely to have affected children because the probability of her marrying another carrier is small if the condition is rare. If the disorder is X-linked the sister of an affected male, who is not the result of a new mutation because his mother is a known carrier, has a 1 in 2 chance of being a carrier and therefore a 1 in 4 chance that any of her sons will also be affected. The demonstration by an appropriate biochemical or other test that *both* parents were carriers of the mutant gene would indicate that the disorder was an autosomal recessive rather than an X-linked trait. In some hereditary disorders there are X-linked and autosomal recessive varieties which can sometimes be distinguished on clinical grounds, as for example in the mucopolysaccharidoses. These are serious diseases characterized by mental retardation, skeletal deformities, and enlargement of the spleen and liver. There are two common forms: an autosomal recessive form (Hurler's syndrome) in which there is defective vision due to clouding of the cornea and an X-linked form (Hunter's syndrome) in which the cornea is clear and vision is unimpaired. Except for this difference these two diseases are almost identical.

GENETIC COUNSELLING AND THE SPORADIC CASE

The distinction between autosomal dominant, autosomal recessive and X-linked modes of inheritance is usually easy and genetic counselling straightforward when there are several affected persons in a family (table XXI). If the condition is rare and there is only one affected person in the family the problem can be very difficult. A common problem arises when normal healthy parents have a child with a rare congenital abnormality and there is no history of anyone else on either side of the family having been similarly

Table XXI. *Proportion of normal and affected progeny of affected parents with different modes of inheritance*

Mode of inheritance	Progeny of affected male		Progeny of heterozygous female	
	Normal	Affected	Normal	Affected
Male Progeny:				
Autosomal recessive	1	0	1	0
Autosomal dominant	1/2	1/2	1/2	1/2
Autosomal dominant (male limited)	1/2	1/2	1/2	1/2
X-linked recessive	1	0	1/2	1/2
X-linked dominant	1	0	1/2	1/2
Female Progeny:				
Autosomal recessive	1	0	1	0
Autosomal dominant	1/2	1/2	1/2	1/2
Autosomal dominant (male limited)	1/2	1/2(c)	1/2	1/2(c)
X-linked recessive	0	1(c)	1/2	1/2(c)
X-linked dominant	0	1	1/2	1/2

(c) indicates a carrier, usually unaffected.

affected. What are the chances that this same abnormality will recur in any future children? There are several possibilities, which are listed below.

1. The condition may not be genetic but due to something the mother was exposed to during her pregnancy (certain drugs, rubella infection, X-irradiation, etc.) (p. 90). In genetic counselling the possibility that a particular congenital abnormality might be the result of some environmental factor must always be borne in mind. The chances that the abnormality will recur in future children will depend on the particular cause. This will be discussed in more detail later.

2. It may be an autosomal dominant condition caused by a new mutation in one of the parents' gametes. If the condition is clearly recognized as one which is always inherited as an autosomal dominant trait and is always fully penetrant (e.g. achondroplasia) and if both parents have been examined and both have been found to be perfectly healthy, then a dominant mutation is the most likely explanation. If such is the case the chance of recurrence in subsequent children is very small.

3. It may be an autosomal recessive disorder. When there is only one affected child in the family, evidence in favour of this being due to a recessive gene would be the demonstration by an appropriate

biochemical or other test that both parents were heterozygotes. Supporting evidence would be if the parents were cousins.

4. It may be an X-linked recessive disorder. This is very unlikely if the affected child is a girl with a normal sex chromosome complement. The distinction between an autosomal recessive and X-linked recessive gene can sometimes be made on clinical grounds as in the case of the mucopolysaccharidoses, and the greater likelihood of one possibility over another depends on the relative incidences of the two forms of the disease. This information is available from published reports in the literature. For example the X-linked form of Duchenne muscular dystrophy is at least 10 times more common than the clinically similar autosomal recessive form of this disease. Quite often with one affected boy in the family it is impossible to decide on the precise mode of inheritance. This is not so important when considering the chances that further children might be affected, because from the practical point of view it is immaterial whether it is autosomal recessive or X-linked. As discussed earlier the distinction is important, however, in advising the sister of an affected male as to whether her children will be affected.

5. Most chromosome abnormalities tend to be sporadic with no one else in the family being affected. Apart from abnormalities of the sex chromosomes, a number of syndromes can now be recognized clinically each of which is associated with a specific chromosome abnormality: Down's syndrome, the 13-trisomy syndrome, the 18-trisomy syndrome, and the cri du chat syndrome (p. 67). A child with abnormalities in more than one system (central nervous system, cardiovascular system, skeletal system, etc.) should always be considered as possibly having a chromosome abnormality and in such cases in order to give genetic counselling advice it is often necessary to study the parents' chromosomes as well on the off-chance that one of the parents carries a translocation. Though families have been described in which several infants have been born with various congenital abnormalities associated with a particular chromosome abnormality, these are the exception rather than the rule. If the parents have normal chromosomes the chances are that the same abnormality will not recur in future children.

6. It may be inherited as a multifactorial trait. Most of these cases occur sporadically and the risks to relatives are usually low (Table XXIII, p. 210).

SOME COMPLICATIONS IN GENETIC COUNSELLING

The rules outlined in the preceding section form a basis for genetic counselling but certain very important considerations should always be borne in mind. We have already mentioned that some hereditary disorders are not always fully penetrant. Occasionally, apparently *normal* parents may have two children who are affected with an autosomal dominant condition. It is extremely unlikely that this could be due to recurrent new mutations and a more likely explanation is that the mutant gene is non-penetrant in one of the parents. Mutations usually affect only a single germ cell but it is possible that a whole section of a gonad may contain the mutant gene (gonadic mosaic) and this would also explain the recurrence of affected offspring to parents who appear to be perfectly healthy. At present, there is no good evidence for gonadic mosaicism in man for any unifactorial disorder. However, mosaicism in a parent can account for the occasional recurrence of chromosome abnormalities in their children.

It is important to know if the condition is variable in its expression. If there is a danger that the condition may occasionally manifest itself in a very severe form this would have to be explained to the parents as well as the chances of recurrence. For example in the condition of cleft hand (lobster claw) the hands and feet may be only slightly deformed, or reduced to pincerlike appendages or so grossly deformed that they are no use at all and have to be amputated. Besides explaining the risks of recurrence to a parent who perhaps is only minimally affected with this condition, it would be necessary to point out that there is a chance that some of his children might be much more severely deformed than he is.

We have mentioned that in genetic counselling every effort should be made to ensure, as far as possible, that the disease in question is not due to some environmental factor (a *phenocopy*). Thus *in utero* infection with toxoplasmosis or cytomegalovirus may produce mental retardation. Certain drugs are known to be teratogenic : thalidomide and limb deformities, aminopterin and CNS malformations, synthetic progestins and abnormal genitalia, chronic alcoholism and mental retardation associated with various congenital malformations, and phenytoin (an anticonvulsant) and cleft palate. Maternal diabetes may be associated with abnormal development of the lower limbs and lumbo-sacral spine. Significant microcephaly is usually defined as a head circumference less that three standard deviations below the mean for any particular age. Thus the head circumference is normally greater than 15 inches (38 cm) at six months, and greater than 16 inches (40·5 cm) at twelve months. Microcephaly with severe mental retardation is often due to a rare recessive gene but may result from X-irradiation of the fetus during pregnancy. Rubella infection during the first three months of pregnancy may cause various abnormalities in the fetus all of which resemble known hereditary conditions. In the case of rubella, surveys have shown that if a pregnant woman contracts the disease during the early weeks of pregnancy there is a 60 per cent chance that her child will be abnormal in some way. The main abnormalities caused by rubella are deafness (in about 50 per cent), congenital heart disease (in just less than 50 per cent) and eye defects (in about 30 per cent). Occasionally the infection may be so mild that the mother may be unaware that she was ever affected. Fortunately there are now serological tests which can detect whether the mother, and more important whether the child, has ever had rubella. If the result is positive in the infant then it is more than likely that the particular malformation is the result of rubella infection rather than the operation of a mutant gene. If this is the case then the abnormality is very unlikely to recur in future children.

A consideration which has to be borne in mind in giving genetic counselling is that conditions which appear very similar on clinical grounds may be inherited in different ways. Different genes which produce apparently identical results are sometimes called *mimic* genes and the phenomenon is referred to as *genetic heterogeneity*. As an example, there are three main forms of muscular dystrophy which all present a similar clinical picture but whereas the Duchenne type is usually inherited as an X-linked recessive, the facio-scapulo-humeral type is inherited as an autosomal dominant and the so-called limb-girdle type is inherited as an autosomal recessive trait. One form of muscle disease, which affects mainly the lower legs and hands (peroneal muscular atrophy) may be inherited as an X-linked recessive, autosomal dominant, or autosomal recessive trait in different families. Clinically there is absolutely no difference between the three conditions. The only difference appears to be the way in which they are inherited and in a small pedigree it might be impossible to distinguish between them. Genetic heterogeneity has been demonstrated in a great many genetic disorders, some of which until recently were considered single diseases. For example there are two types of complete albinism (tyrosinase positive and tyrosinase negative) and haematological studies indicate that there are at least three and possibly four different types of haemophilia. It is probable that the majority of genetic disorders will be found to be heterogenous when adequately investigated by appropriate methods.

Another phenomenon has recently been described which may complicate genetic counselling. A person affected with a recessive disorder will not have affected children, except in the rare event of marrying a carrier of the same disease. In the case of a rare disorder such as phenylketonuria this is extremely unlikely. However, several cases have been reported recently of women with phenylketonuria who have married normal men but have had children with severe mental retardation. It seems that the explanation has nothing to do with genetic mechanisms but is the result of the fetus being damaged by high concentrations of some metabolite which traverses the placenta from the mother to the fetus during pregnancy. The children do not have the genetic biochemical defect but their brains are nevertheless damaged in the same way as children who do have the disease.

Many individuals with phenylketonuria who have been success-fully treated with phenylalanine-free diets will be reaching child-bearing age within the next few years. The possibility of their child-ren being mentally retarded will have to be considered. Authorities on this disease differ as to exactly how long a child with phenyl-ketonuria should be kept on a phenylalanine-restricted diet. Some believe that a normal diet can be introduced by the age of 3 without causing any harm. The observations on phenylketonuric women who have had mentally retarded children indicate that a phenylalanine-restricted diet may have to be reintroduced when a phenylketonuric mother becomes pregnant if damage to the fetal brain is to be prevented.

COUSIN MARRIAGES

In the ancient royal families of Egypt it was customary for cousins or even brothers and sisters to marry each other in order to keep the royal blood 'pure'. It is doubtful if such a system would have been retained if it had led to any marked increase in congenital abnorma-lities in the children of such matches. However, several extensive studies have shown that among the offspring of consanguineous marriages there is an increased post-natal mortality rate and an increased frequency of congenital abnormalities and mental retarda-tion, but the actual risks are small and many couples will accept them.

The situation is quite different if there is a history of recessive disorder in the family. The chance of first cousins carrying the same gene is 1 in 8. Therefore if there is a family history of a recessive disorder, such as phenylketonuria, then the chance of two cousins having affected offspring is considerably greater than in the case of unrelated parents. If, for example, two cousins have an uncle with phenylketonuria then the chance of their having an affected child is about 1 in 36 whereas the chance of two unrelated persons having an affected child is about 1 in 10,000. The figures are arrived at in the following way. If two cousins have an affected uncle (or aunt) the chance of their parents being carriers is $\frac{2}{3}$ and thus the chance that the cousins themselves are carriers is $\frac{2}{6}$. The chance of any child of such a cousin marriage being affected is therefore $\frac{2}{6} \times \frac{2}{6} \times \frac{1}{4} = \frac{1}{36}$. Since the frequency of carriers of phenylketonuria in the general population is about 1 in 50 the chance that two unrelated persons will have an affected child is $\frac{1}{50} \times \frac{1}{50} \times \frac{1}{4} = \frac{1}{10000}$. Cousin marriages not only have an increased risk of producing a child homozygous for a detrimental recessive gene but also of producing a child with a disorder due to many genes.

In summary, if cousins marry the chance that they will have a child with some congenital abnormality is little greater than in the general population. If, however, someone in the family is affected with a disorder caused either by many genes or by a single recessive gene, then the chance of first cousins having an affected child is much greater than in the general population, and in such circumstances having children would be inadvisable.

Several studies have shown that at least one-third of children of unions between close relatives (incest) have severe congenital malformations and are mentally retarded. According to ancient canon law it was forbidden for a man or woman to have intercourse with various relatives (see Leviticus chap 18), but most of these strictures had no genetic foundation. Today the law relating to incest (Sexual Offences Act, 1956) is more meaningful since it forbids a man to have intercourse with his grand-daughter and any first-degree female relatives, and for a woman to give consent to have intercourse with her grand-father and any first-degree male relatives.

Chromosome Studies and Genetic Counselling

Chromosome studies are used in genetic counselling in cases of abnormal sexual development, infertility, recurrent abortion, and in infants with congenital defects where the clinician suspects that the cause is a chromosome aberration.

Advances in human cytogenetics have completely changed the physician's approach to problems involving abnormalities of sexual development. Today his first concern is to exclude a chromosome abnormality as the possible cause. For example, a young woman who has reached the age of about 20 but has not yet begun to menstruate and whose breasts have not developed may have either Turner's syndrome, or an endocrine abnormality, or merely delayed puberty. A buccal smear, if chromatin negative, would suggest that she is a case of Turner's syndrome and this could be verified by chromosome studies. The finding of a chromosomal abnormality would mean that further investigations are unnecessary. On the other hand, if the condition was due to an endocrine abnormality, very extensive investigations would have to be undertaken in order to define the precise nature of the hormonal disturbance so that appropriate therapy might be given.

An increasing number of cases of infertility are being referred for chromosome studies since an occasional cause is a sex chromosomal abnormality in one of the partners. In males with infertility for which there is no apparent endocrinological or anatomical cause, about 7 per cent prove to have Klinefelter's syndrome and 3 per cent have morphological rearrangements of the Y chromosome or sex chromosome mosaicism. Therapeutic measures designed to increase fertility in such patients' are valueless and AID (artificial insemination by donor) or child adoption might have to be considered by the husband and wife.

About 15 per cent of all conceptions terminate in either a spontaneous abortion or a stillbirth. It has been appreciated for many years that spontaneous abortions may occur in women who are badly nourished or in poor health and it is well known that anatomical abnormalities of the uterus and certain endocrine abnormalities in the mother may lead to the fetus being aborted. However, there is growing evidence that the factor causing embryonic death may sometimes be inherent in the embryo itself. In an extensive investigation of the chromosomes in spontaneous abortions, Carr found chromosomal aberrations in more than 20 per cent of the fetuses. Many of these chromosomal abnormalities, which include autosomal monosomy and triploidy, have not been found in live-born babies and are therefore presumably lethal. Others, such as XO, are sometimes compatible with survival (p. 70). The risk of recurrence in these types of abnormalities is small. Nevertheless, sometimes in cases of recurrent abortion one of the parents carries a translocation which in the unbalanced state in the fetus is lethal. The parent who carries the translocation has the normal amount of genetic material and is therefore perfectly healthy. The situation is similar to that in some cases of Down's syndrome except that in these the genetic imbalance in the fetus (46 chromosomes with a D/G translocation) is not lethal. Depending on the particular type of chromosomal rearrangement found in the carrier parent the risks of further abortions may be very high. In some instances it might be predicted that no live births would be possible. So far not enough cases have been studied for us to know the proportion of spontaneous abortions which are due to one of the parents being a carrier of a translocation or other chromosome abnormality. Certainly there seems good reason to carry out chromosome studies on both parents in those cases of recurrent abortion where the cause is not obvious. In one investigation chromosome studies were reported in 228 married couples with repeated abortions and in 30 of these couples (13 per cent) some abnormality of the karyotype was found in one of the spouses (Käosaar & Mikelsaar, 1973).

Besides chromosome aberrations, recurrent abortion may be due to an immune reaction on the part of the group O mother to a fetus which is blood group A or B. Her antibodies to A and B blood-group substances traverse the placenta and may lead to fetal death if they are of sufficiently high concentration (titre). For this reason investigations of cases of recurrent abortion might usefully include blood-group studies on the parents including an estimation of the titre of blood-group antibodies in the mother's serum. It is also important to bear in mind that abortions may represent lethal equivalents of certain postnatal anomalies. This has been postulated in central nervous system malformations such as congenital hydrocephalus.

The use of chromosome studies in infants with congenital abnormalities has already been referred to. Such studies have proved particularly valuable in the case of translocation Down's syndrome where it has been found that the risks of recurrence in future children depend on the type of translocation (table XXII). Cytologically it is now possible to distinguish between a 21/21 and 21/22 translocation. The distinction is important because the risk of recurrence in the former is 100 per cent whereas in the latter it is only about 1 in 20. We saw earlier that the *theoretical* risk of a mother with a D/G translocation having an affected child is about 1 in 3. In fact, for reasons which are still not clear, the *actual* risk is probably less, being about 1 in 10. If the father is the translocation carrier the risk of having an affected child is only about 1 in 20 (table XXII). The preferential transmission of translocation trisomic offspring by female rather than male translocation carriers have also been described in mouse which may therefore make a useful model for studying this phenomenon (Eicher, 1973).

ADOPTION AND DISPUTED PATERNITY

The physician interested in genetics is often called upon to answer problems involving child adoption. The questions usually come from adoption agencies who wish to place a child but are reluctant to do so because of some disorder in the child's background suspected of being hereditary. In many cases complete reassurance is possible; the main difficulties arise when there is a family history of a disease which is not recognizable clinically or biochemically during the first year of life. This is so for example in Marfan's syndrome (tall, thin

Table XXII. *Recurrence risk of Down's syndrome due to various chromosome aberrations.*

	Karyotypes		Chance of recurrence %
Patient	Father	Mother	
Translocation:			
D/G	N	C	10
	C	N	5
21/22	N	C	7
	C	N	<3
21/21	C	N	100
	N	C	100
Trisomy-21	N	N	1
Translocation or mosaic	N	N	small

C=carrier; N=normal.

patients with long tapering fingers and toes, dislocation of the lens of the eye, and rupture of the aorta), and the adult type of polycystic kidney disease. Advances in biochemistry may soon enable us to recognize preclinical cases of such diseases and thus to deal with them more adequately.

Disputed paternity is a thorny problem in which the medical geneticist sometimes becomes involved. It is a golden rule that paternity can never be *proved* with absolute certainty but can be disproved in two ways. First, if a child is found to possess a blood-group substance not present in either of its parents, then the putative father cannot be the true father. Second, if the child lacks a blood-group substance which the putative father would have had to transmit to any of his offspring. For example, if the mother and the putative father lack blood group B yet the child has that blood group then the true father must have had it, and a putative father with blood group AB cannot have a child with blood group O.

GENETIC COUNSELLING IN COMMON
DISEASES—EMPIRIC RISKS

There are a certain number of fairly common conditions in which heredity plays an important part but where there is no simple mode of inheritance. Some of these conditions are probably heterogeneous and include a number of aetiologically different disorders; others are probably due to many genes and also the effect of environment. In such conditions as these the risks of recurrence are empirical. The term *empiric risk* may be defined as the probability of occurrence of a specified event based upon prior experience and observation rather than on prediction by a general theory (Herndon, 1962). Empiric risks are determined by estimating the frequency of the condition in the relatives of affected persons.

Approximate empiric risk figures for some common conditions are given in table XXIII. The risks apply only to conditions which are not inherited in any simple manner. For instance, mental retardation may be inherited as a recessive trait in which case the risk of recurrence in sibs is 25 per cent. However, many cases of mental retardation are not inherited in any simple manner and in these cases the risk of recurrence in sibs is about 3 to 5 per cent.

In multifactorial disorders the rate of recurrence in first-degree relatives is approximately equal to the square root of the prevalence in the general population. Since the prevalence of most multifactorial disorders is between 1 in 500 and 1 in 2000 the recurrence rate is usually between 2 and 5 per cent.

Unfortunately empiric risk figures are rarely available for situations where there are several affected members in a family or for disorders with variable severity and different sex incidences. A computer program is available in which all these factors can be included in estimating recurrence risks (Smith, 1972).

CARRIER RECOGNITION

If we were able to recognize carriers of autosomal recessive traits, X-linked recessive traits, and non-penetrant autosomal dominant traits much doubt and uncertainty would be removed from genetic counselling. During the last few years the detection of genetic carriers has become one of the most important fields of research in medical genetics.

In some conditions carriers can be recognized with a high degree of certainty. This is so in acatalasia, a condition in which there is a deficiency in the blood of the enzyme catalase which breaks down hydrogen peroxide (p. 142). In the other diseases only a proportion of

carriers can be detected as in the case of haemophilia, phenylketonuria, and galactosaemia. In other conditions no method has yet been
found which will distinguish carriers. This is so, for example, in
alkaptonuria.

There are several possible ways in which carriers of genetic
diseases might be recognized. Occasionally they may have some of

Table XXIII. *Empiric risks for some common disorders (in per cent)*

Disorder	Incidence	Sex ratio M : F	Normal parents having a second affected child	Affected parent having an affected child	Affected parent having a second affected child
Anencephaly	0·20	1 : 2	2	—	—
Cleft palate only	0·04	2 : 3	2	7	15
Cleft lip ± cleft palate	0·10	3 : 2	4	4	10
Club foot	0·10	2 : 1	3	3	10
Cong. heart disease (all types)	0·50	—	1–4	1–4	—
Diabetes mellitus (early onset)	0·20	1 : 1	8	8	10
Dislocation of hip	0·07	1 : 6	4	4	10
Epilepsy (' idiopathic ')	0·50	1 : 1	5	5	10
Hirschsprung's disease	0·02	4 : 1			
male index			2	—	—
female index			8	—	—
Manic-depressive psychoses	0·40	2 : 3	—	10–15	—
Mental retardation (' idiopathic ')	0·30 −0·50	1 : 1	3–5	—	—
Profound childhood deafness	0·10	1 : 1	10	6	—
Pyloric stenosis	0·30	5 : 1			
male index			2	4	13
female index			10	17	38
Schizophrenia	1–2	1 : 1	—	16	—
Scoliosis (idiopathic, adolescent)	0·22	1 : 6	7	5	—
Spina bifida	0·30	2 : 3	4	3	—

the clinical manifestations of the disease. These manifestations are
usually so slight that they are only obvious on very careful clinical
examination. Such manifestations, even though minimal, may be
unmistakably pathological as in the case of X-linked ocular albinism.
Unfortunately in many conditions there are either no manifestations at all in the carrier or they are so slight as to be misinter-

preted as normal variations. This is so in some carriers of haemophilia who have a tendency to bruise easily, but this of course can occur in perfectly normal women. Thus clinical manifestations are only of importance in detecting carriers when they are unmistakably pathological, and in most conditions this is rare.

The demonstration of linkage between an hereditary disorder and one of the marker traits would be of great help in carrier recognition, particularly if the gene were so close to the marker trait that crossing-over very rarely occurred. This would be especially valuable in the case of X-linked disorders. In a particular family, if each affected hemizygous male were known to have the marker trait, the demonstration of this trait in a female in the same family would suggest that she was a carrier of the disease. Unfortunately none of the X-linked marker traits are sufficiently close to any of the serious X-linked disorders to be of any practical value in carrier recognition. So far, the results of autosomal linkage studies have also been rather unhelpful though the recent findings of linkage between one form of congenital cataract and the Duffy blood-group locus may prove useful in genetic counselling (p. 52).

With regard to carrier detection, by far the most important discovery in recent years has been the demonstration of detectable biochemical abnormalities in carriers of certain diseases. In some diseases the biochemical abnormality is a *direct* result of gene action in the heterozygous state. This is so in carriers of acatalasia. As we saw earlier, certain individuals with this condition have no catalase in their blood; in carriers the amount of enzyme is intermediate between levels found in normal persons and affected persons. Often the biochemical abnormality which is detectable in the carrier is not a direct result of gene action but is the result of some secondary process. *We are less able to recognize the carrier state the farther we are from the primary action of the mutant gene.* For example, in Duchenne muscular dystrophy, the primary cause is unknown but a comparatively early manifestation of the disease is an increased permeability of the muscle membrane and an escape of muscular enzymes into the blood. *Later* the muscle fibres undergo degeneration and are replaced by fatty connective tissue and as a consequence in the later stages of the disease increased amounts of creatine are excreted in the urine. In carriers of this disease only a small proportion have been found to excrete excessive amounts of creatine in their urine and as a consequence this test could not be used to detect carriers. However, over 60 per cent of carriers have an elevated serum level of creatine kinase, one of the enzymes which leaks out of the muscle into the blood (table XXIV).

The investigation of carriers may lead not only to reliable tests for the identification of such carriers but may help our understanding of the pathogenesis of a particular disease. Abnormalities only detectable in affected individuals are probably farther from the primary action of the gene than abnormalities found in apparently perfectly healthy carriers.

With rare diseases carrier detection is most important in families in which affected cases are known to have occurred and is particularly important in the case of X-linked conditions, for example, in

Table XXIV. *Carrier detection in X-linked disorders*

Disorder	Abnormality
Haemophilia A	factor VIII reduced*
Haemophilia B	factor IX reduced
G-6-PD deficiency	erythrocyte G-6-PD reduced
Congenital agammaglobulinaemia	*in vitro* immunoglobulin synthesis by lymphocytes reduced
Lesch-Nyhan syndrome	hypoxanthine-guanine phosphoribosyl transferase in skin fibroblasts reduced. Two populations of cells
Hunter's syndrome	accumulation of sulphate in skin fibroblasts. Two populations of cells
Ocular albinism	patchy depigmentation of retina and iris
Vit. D resistant rickets (hypophosphataemia)	serum phosphorous reduced
Duchenne muscular dystrophy	serum creatine kinase raised
Becker muscular dystrophy	serum creatine kinase raised
Diabetes insipidus (nephrogenic)	urine concentration diminished
Fabry's disease (angiokeratoma)	α-galactosidase in skin fibroblasts reduced. Two populations of cells
Chronic granulomatous disease (one type)	leucocyte phagocytosis and nitro blue tetrazolium test abnormal
Retinitis pigmentosa	tapetal reflex
Anhidrotic ectodermal dysplasia	sweat pore counts reduced

* More precisely a reduction in the ratio of factor VIII activity to inactive antigen.

counselling the sister of a man with haemophilia. Carrier detection has relatively little practical application in the case of rare autosomal recessive traits. However, in common diseases due to recessive genes population surveys may be useful in detecting carriers who could then be warned of the risk of having affected children if they marry each other. Already such investigations are being undertaken in parts of Italy where 10 per cent or more of the population carry the gene for thalassaemia. This disease, it will be remembered, is due to an autosomal recessive gene which in homozygous form produces a profound and usually fatal anaemia (p. 37). The only condition in Europe and the United States in which such large-scale public health measures might find application is in the case of fibrocystic disease of the pancreas. About 4 per cent of Europeans carry the gene responsible for this disease, but unfortunately as yet there is no reliable method for detecting carriers. Incidentally though comparatively common in Europeans, phenylketonuria and fibrocystic disease are relatively uncommon in Africans.

ACCEPTABILITY OF GENETIC RISKS

When parents prove to be carriers of a detrimental mutant gene or a chromosome abnormality their decision as to whether or not to have further children is influenced by the severity of the abnormality, whether there is an effective treatment, the actual risk, their religious attitudes, socio-economic status and education.

From the foregoing discussions it will be seen that the risks of recurrence for hereditary diseases vary considerably from as high as 100 per cent in the case of parents homozygous for the same recessive gene, down to 2 per cent in certain congenital abnormalities. We may therefore ask ourselves, 'What is an acceptable risk?' It is difficult to give a simple answer to this question. It will largely depend on the severity of the condition. A 50 per cent risk of developing syndactyly (fused fingers and toes) a condition which is readily amenable to surgery and causes little inconvenience may be acceptable, but some people might find a risk of 4 per cent unacceptable in a condition such as spina bifida. It will depend on the parents' attitude to the disease and their socio-economic background. It may be considerably easier for a wealthy couple to care for a paralysed child than for less fortunate parents. It is sometimes consoling to know that about 2 per cent of all live births have some abnormality and most parents are willing to accept a risk of 10 per cent or less. After all this means that there is a 90 per cent or more chance that their children will *not be* affected.

The decision to have further children is usually left to the parents. The medical geneticist merely explains the risks and makes every effort to remove any feelings of guilt which might be present. However, in one study (Carter, 1970) about a third of high risk families planned further children after genetic counselling despite the risks involved. This suggests that perhaps the genetic counsellor, at least in the case of serious genetic disorders with a high risk of recurrence, might feel obliged to do more than merely explain the risks and suggest that family limitation would be advisable. Further, recent follow-up studies indicate that parents are influenced as much by the ' burden ' of an affected child on the family as they are by the actual risks of recurrence (Emery *et al.*, 1973), and therefore it is important to discuss the prognosis and availability of treatment.

ANTENATAL DIAGNOSIS OF GENETIC DISEASE

Contraception is not the only course of action open to parents who are at risk of having a child with a serious genetic disorder (table XXV). Other possibilities include sterilization, and artificial insemination by donor (AID) in cases where both parents are heterozygous for the same *rare* recessive trait, or the father is affected with a dominant or X-linked disorder.

Table XXV. *Possibilities open to parents who have had a child with a particular disorder, or are themselves affected (e.g. osteogenesis imperfecta) or carry a particular chromosome translocation (Down's syndrome)*

Example	risk (%)	contra-ception	steril-ization	abortion
Cleft palate alone	2	—	—	—
Spina bifida (1 affected child)	4	?	—	—*
Spina bifida (2 affected children)	10	+	?	? *
Galactosaemia	25	+	+	+ *
Duchenne muscular dystrophy	50 (sons)	+	+	+
	50 (daughters)			
Osteogenesis imperfecta	50	+	+	+
Down's syndrome				
D/G translocation	5–10	+	+	+ *
21/21 translocation	100	+	+	+

*Antenatal diagnosis possible.

With the liberalization of the Abortion Law in 1968 termination of pregnancy is possible if there is a ' substantial risk ' of a serious abnormality in the fetus. Recently *selective* abortion has also become possible whereby a pregnancy need only be terminated when the fetus is *known* to be abnormal. Antenatal diagnosis with selective abortion of an abnormal fetus is becoming an accepted procedure in the management of families at high risk of producing a child with serious hereditary disorder (see Emery, 1973). This is possible by removing a small volume (5-10 ml) of amniotic fluid by aspiration through the abdominal wall (transabdominal amniocentesis) around the fourteenth week of gestation. The cells contained in the amniotic fluid are of fetal origin being derived from fetal skin and amnion. Most of these cells are dead squames but a small proportion are viable and will grow in tissue culture. Uncultured cells may be used to sex the fetus from X- and Y-chromatin studies. In this way a woman at high risk of having a son with a serious X-linked disorder can be guaranteed a daughter who will not be affected but of course will have half the risk her mother has of also being a carrier. Since by this technique sons will be replaced by daughters, a proportion of whom will be carriers, the result will be to produce an increase in the number of carriers in the population. A more efficient way of reducing the frequency of X-linked genes in the population would be the selective abortion of female fetuses of fathers with such disorders as haemophilia or Becker muscular dystrophy since all their daughters must be carriers but all their sons will be normal. In this way, except for new mutations, the incidence of such disorders could be reduced considerably. The only way in which the incidence of affected males *and* carrier females could be reduced would be when both hemizygous affected males and carrier females can be detected *in utero* (as is the case in Lesch-Nyhan syndrome) and parents decide to have only normal sons and daughters, all affected males or carrier females being aborted.

Sexing of the fetus based on the study of uncultured cells is not reliable and in doubtful cases it is better to study the karyotype of *cultured* cells. After centrifugation of the amniotic fluid specimen, the button of cells is resuspended in culture medium such as Eagle's minimum essential medium with 30 per cent fetal calf serum. After ten to fourteen days there are usually sufficient cells for chromosome studies though it may be several weeks before there are sufficient cells for biochemical studies. The most frequent chromosomal abnormality where amniocentesis is indicated is when there is a risk of having a child with Down's syndrome. This risk may be as high as 1 in 100 in women who have previously had a child with trisomy-21, 1 in 50 in women over the age of 40 and at least 1 in 20 if one of the parents carries a D/G translocation (see p. 208). So far some sixty inborn errors of metabolism can be diagnosed *in utero* from a study of cultured amniotic fluid cells. They include galactosaemia, Hunter's and Hurler's syndromes, homocystinuria, Lesch-Nyhan syndrome, maple syrup urine disease and Tay-Sachs' disease. Disorders in which the specific enzyme deficiency cannot be demonstrated in epithelial tissues, but only in other tissues (e.g. phenylalanine hydroxylase activity is only present in liver cells), cannot therefore be detected *in utero* by this means (e.g.

phenylketonuria). It is also not possible to diagnose fibrocystic disease *in utero* since in this disorder the primary enzyme defect has not yet been identified.

Finally, from measurements of alphafetoprotein levels in amniotic fluid it is now possible to detect anencephaly and open spina bifida *in utero* in early pregnancy. There is a suggestion that the antenatal diagnosis of such disorders may also be possible from measuring levels of alphafetoprotein in maternal serum since this is often raised when amniotic fluid levels are raised.

At one time it was believed that the β chain of adult haemoglobin was synthesized by the fetus only towards term. However, there is now evidence which indicates that β chain synthesis is demonstrable as early as 12 weeks' gestation. Since the defect in sickle-cell anaemia resides in the β chain (p. 33) this opens up the possibility of diagnosing this disorder *in utero* provided specimens of fetal blood can be obtained. Recently it has been reported that this is possible by inserting a needle into the umbilical vessels under direct vision through a fetoscope. Further uses of such a fetoscope would be in diagnosing *in utero* congenital malformations (such as lobster claw deformity) not associated with any specific chromosomal or biochemical defect.

TREATMENT OF GENETIC DISEASE

It is often assumed that once the diagnosis of genetic disease has been made, little more can be done for the patient. This is not true. The recognition of the basic biochemical defect can lead to the development of effective methods of treatment, though *cure,* in the sense of replacing a mutant gene by a normal gene, seems a very remote possibility at present. Examples of some hereditary diseases which illustrate various approaches to treatment are given in table XXVI. Most of these disorders have already been mentioned in previous chapters. Methylmalonic-acidaemia and propionicacidaemia are rare recessive disorders associated with failure to thrive and severe metabolic disturbances. Argininaemia is associated with mental retardation as are some cases of cystathioninuria. Trypsinogen deficiency results in hypoproteinaemia and failure to thrive.

When a disorder is due to an enzyme block then the defective enzyme or protein might be replaced or its substrate restricted or the deficient product can be replaced. The replacement of a deficient coenzyme is also effective in some disorders. Unfortunately most hereditary metabolic disorders involve enzymes which have not been isolated or synthesized. Injection of these enzymes, even if available, might not be effective because many perform their catalytic function

Table XXVI. *Examples of various methods for treating genetic disease.* P= *possible but not yet proven.* S= *effective in some cases*

Therapy	Disorder
1 *Enzyme induction*:	
(a) by virus	
Shope virus (P)	argininaemia
(b) by drugs	
phenobarbitone	cong. nonhaemolytic jaundice
2 *Replacement of deficient enzyme*:	
(a) tissue transplantation (S)	Fabry's disease
(b) enzyme preps: trypsin	trypsinogen deficiency
(c) plasma or leucocyte infusions (P)	mucopolysaccharidoses
3 *Replacement of deficient protein*:	
antihaemophilic globulin	haemophilia
4 *Replacement of deficient vitamin or coenzyme*:	
B6	cystathioninuria
B12	methylmalonicacidaemia (S)
biotin	propionicacidaemia (S)
D	vit. D resistant rickets
5 *Replacement of deficient product*:	
cortisone	adrenogenital syndrome
cysteine	homocystinuria
thyroxine	cong. cretinism
uridine	oroticaciduria
6 *Substrate restriction in diet*:	
(a) aminoacids	
phenylalanine	phenylketonuria
leucine, isoleucine and valine	maple syrup urine disease
methionine	homocystinuria
(b) carbohydrate	
galactose	galactosaemia
(c) lipid	
cholesterol	hypercholesterolaemia
7 *Drug therapy*:	
aminocaproic acid	angioneurotic oedema
cholestyramine	hypercholesterolaemia
insulin	diabetes
pancreatin	fibrocystic disease
penicillamine	Wilson's disease
8 *Preventive therapy*:	
avoidance of certain drugs	G6PD deficiency, porphyria
Rh gamma globulin	Rh incompatibility
9 *Replacement of defective tissues*:	
kidney transplantation	polycystic kidney disease
corneal graft	cong. keratoconus
10 *Removal of diseased tissues*:	
colectomy	polyposis coli
splenectomy	hereditary spherocytosis
neurofibromata	neurofibromatosis
11 *Portacaval anastomosis*	hepatic glycogenoses
	hyperlipoproteinaemia

within cells. In these cases replacement of a defective enzyme by the transplantation of tissue possessing normal enzyme activity might be a possibility in the future. Recently it has been suggested that the treatment of certain genetic disorders may be possible by the infusion of normal plasma or leucocytes which replace an enzyme which is deficient in the disorder in question. This approach has been of some success in the case of certain mucopolysaccharidoses.

When a genetic disease is due to a mutation of a control gene so that the synthesis of a specific enzyme is merely 'switched off', drug therapy might be effective by inducing enzyme synthesis. This is now possible in the case of congenital nonhaemolytic jaundice in which the enzyme glucuronyl transferase can be induced by treatment with small doses of phenobarbitone. It has recently been suggested that since the Shope papilloma virus of rabbits induces the synthesis of the enzyme arginase without having any adverse effect when injected into humans, this might be an effective treatment for argininaemia. This could be considered an example of *genetic engineering*, i.e. the treatment of genetic disease by actually altering the DNA of the patient. There are considerable scientific and ethical problems associated with such an approach to treatment (Friedmann and Roblin, 1972) and as yet it remains within the realms of speculation. Nevertheless the possibility may not be too far ahead, for Merril and his colleagues have shown that the enzyme deficiency in fibroblasts in culture from a patient with galactosaemia can be corrected by infection with a particular bacteriophage (lambda phage from *E. coli*) which carries the missing gene. Whether or not a phage can ever be used as a vehicle for introducing a selected gene into human cells *in vivo* as a means of treatment is, however, an open question.

Drug therapy can also be effective in certain disorders. For example, cholestyramine lowers the serum level of cholesterol and the effect on patients with hypercholesterolaemia is now being investigated. Penicillamine increases the urinary excretion of copper and is proving beneficial in the treatment of patients with Wilson's disease.

Preventative therapy, surgical removal of diseased tissue and transplantation with normal tissue are more obvious ways of treating certain genetic diseases.

In summary, genetic disease need not be approached with a sense of therapeutic inadequacy. There are many disorders at present for which effective therapy is available and no doubt the list will increase as more is learned of the basic biochemical abnormalities underlying hereditary disorders.

FUTURE POSSIBILITIES

We might end by mentioning some future possibilities in medical genetics. Apart from the obvious problem of finding effective treatments for genetic disorders, there is an important need to ensure that genetic advice is made as widely available as possible. There is evidence that there are many people in the population who are at risk of having a child with a serious hereditary disorder but are unaware of this. Increasing knowledge of genetics and appreciation of the risks by physicians will help to reduce this problem. There is however, an important need to set up *genetic registers* in which families with serious hereditary disorders are recorded so that individuals at high risk in these families can be carefully followed up and given appropriate counselling. In Edinburgh such a register has already been developed and is referred to by the acronym *RAPID: R*egister for the *A*scertainment and *P*revention of *I*nherited *D*isease, the main function of which is the prevention of genetic disease (Emery *et al.*, 1974).

Associated with the problem of recognizing carriers is that of recognizing *preclinical* cases and those who are genetically predisposed to particular diseases. Infants with phenylketonuria are treated as soon as possible before clinical signs of the disease have had time to develop, and we mentioned earlier the recent interest in recognizing and treating prediabetics in order to prevent the disease from developing later in life. In families with polyposis coli persons at risk should undergo regular sigmoidoscopy, and there is good reason for considering colectomy in those who develop polyps because of the very real danger of malignant change occurring.

At some future time when we are able to recognize persons predisposed to such a disease as schizophrenia it may be possible to prevent the disease either by suitable drugs or even by special psychotherapy. One day there may even be a place for treating the child with a hereditary disorder *before* birth. Recent work with mice makes this suggestion appear a little less remote than it at first seems. In mice there is a particular eye defect which leads to blindness and is caused by an autosomal recessive gene. If pregnant female mice are treated with cortisone, this eye anomaly in their offspring can be prevented. Similarly in certain strains of mice thyroxine administered to pregnant females reduces the incidence of spontaneously occurring hare lip and dietary supplements of manganese given to the mother during pregnancy prevents hereditary ataxia in certain other strains. This is not meant to imply that these findings suggest cures for analogous diseases in man but they do indicate another way in which the prevention of genetic disease might be approached in the future. There are already reports that it may be possible to prevent congenital non-haemolytic jaundice by giving mothers small doses of phenobarbitone before delivery, and the respiratory distress syndrome, which is prevalent in premature infants can be prevented by giving the mother certain steroids before delivery. Familial pyridoxine dependent congenital epilepsy (a recessive disorder) can be prevented if the mother is given pyridoxine daily during the latter part of pregnancy. Finally, recent work on mice suggests that it might be possible to mitigate the expression of Pendred syndrome (a recessive disorder characterised by congenital deafness and hypothyroidism) by giving thyroxine during pregnancy.

Exchange blood transfusions have been given successfully to rhesus (Rh) negative babies while *in utero* and Professor Clarke's group in Liverpool have even gone one step further in their attempt to prevent Rh incompatibility. It appears that when a baby is born some of its cells find their way into the mother's circulation via the placenta. If the child is Rh positive and the mother Rh negative she will react by producing Rh antibodies to the fetal cells. When next she becomes pregnant, if the fetus is Rh positive the maternal antibodies will damage the fetus. One way of preventing sensitization and therefore Rh incompatibility is to inject Rh antibodies into the mother shortly after delivery so that any fetal cells which have found their way into the maternal circulation might be destroyed before they have had time to sensitize the mother. Results so far are most encouraging. However, such an approach is no use when the mother has already become immunized against the Rh antigen. In this situation maternal antibody may be removed by plasmapheresis. This technique along with the giving of Rh gamma globulin may soon remove the problem of rhesus sensitization completely.

In the future the physician may become more involved in treating people who appear perfectly healthy but are genetically predisposed to a particular disease. He may even find himself treating mothers during pregnancy in order to prevent certain hereditary diseases in their offspring. Medical genetics seems likely to become the preventive medicine of the future.

FURTHER READING

Beighton, P. and Nelson, M. M. (1974). Medical genetics in clinical practice. *S.A. Med. J.* **48,** 1759-1762.
Carr, D. H. (1963). Chromosome studies in abortuses and stillborn infants. *Lancet*, **2,** 603-606.
Carter, C. O. (1970). Prospects in genetic counselling. In *Modern Trends in Human Genetics*. Vol. 1. Ed. Emery, A. E. H. pp. 339-349. London : Butterworths.

Carter, C. O. and Evans, K. (1973). Children of adult survivors with spina bifida cystica. *Lancet,* **2,** 924-926.

Childs, B. and Young, W. J. (1963). Genetic variations in man. *Am J. Med.* **34,** 663-673.

Clarke, C. A., Elson, C. J., Bradley, J., Donohue, W. T. A. and Lehane, D. (1970). Intensive plasmapheresis as a therapeutic measure in rhesus-immunized women. *Lancet,* **1,** 793-798.

Clow, C. L., Fraser, F. C., Laberge, C. and Scriver, C. R. (1973). On the application of knowledge to the patient with genetic disease. *Prog. med. Genet.* **9,** 159-213.

Crigler, J. F. (1969). Phenobarbital, hormones and bilirubin. *Johns Hopkins med. J.* **125,** 245-249.

Eicher, E. M. (1973). Translocation trisomic mice. *Science,* **180,** 81.

Emery, A. E. H. (1969). Genetic counselling. *Scott. med. J.* **14,** 335-347.

Emery, A. E. H. (1973). *Antenatal Diagnosis of Genetic Disease.* Edinburgh: Churchill Livingstone.

Emery, A. E. H., Watt, M. S. and Clack, E. R. (1973). Social effects of genetic counselling. *Brit. med. J.* **1,** 724-726.

Emery, A. E. H. et al. (1974). A genetic register system (*RAPID*). *J. Med. Genet.* **11,** 145-151.

Friedmann, T. and Roblin, R. (1972). Gene therapy for human genetic disease. *Science,* **175,** 949-955.

Finn, R. (1970). The prevention of Rh haemolytic disease. In *Modern Trends in Human Genetics.* Vol. 1. Ed. Emery, A. E. H. pp. 297-315. London : Butterworths.

Hamerton, J. L. (1968). Robertsonian translocation in man: evidence for prezygotic selection. *Cytogenetics,* **7,** 260-276.

Herndon, C. N. (1962). Empiric risks. In *Methodology in Human Genetics.* Ed. Burdette, W. J., pp. 144-155. San Francisco: Holden-Day.

Heuch, I. and Li, F. H. F. (1972). *PEDIG*—a computer program for calculation of genotype probabilities using phenotype information. *Clin. Genet.* **3,** 501-504.

Hsia, D. Y. Y. (1969). The detection of heterozygous carriers. *Med. Clins N. Am.* **53,** 857-874.

Jones, K. L., et al. (1974). Outcome in offspring of chronic alcoholic women. *Lancet,* **1,** 1076-1078.

Käosaar, M. E. and Mikelsaar, A-V. N. (1973). Chromosome investigation in married couples with repeated spontaneous abortions. *Humangenetik,* **17,** 277-283.

Lynch, H. T., Krush, T. P. and Krush, A. J. et al. (1964). Psychodynamics of early hereditary deaths. Role of the medical genetics counselor. *Am. J. Dis. Child.* **108,** 605-610.

Merril, C. R., Geier, M. R. and Petricciani, J. C. (1971). Bacterial virus gene expression in human cells. *Nature, Lond.* **233,** 398-400.

Motulsky, A. G. and Gartler, S. M. (1959). Consanguinity and marriage. *Practitioner,* **183,** 170-177.

Motulsky, A. G. and Hecht, F. (1964). Genetic prognosis and counseling. *Am. J. Obstet. Gynec.* **90,** 1227-1241.

Murphy, E. A. (1968). The rationale of genetic counseling. *J. Pediat.* **72,** 121-130.

Murphy, E. A. (1970). The ' Ensu ' scoring system in genetic counselling. *Ann. hum. Genet.* **34,** 73-78.

Nadler, H. L. (1969). Prenatal detection of genetic defects. *J. Pediat.* **74,** 132–143.

Richardson, D. W. (1975). Artificial insemination in the human. In *Modern Trends in Human Genetics.* Vol. 2. Ed. Emery, A. E. H. pp. 404–448. London: Butterworths.

Roberts, D. F., Chavez, J. and Court, S. D. M. (1970). The genetic component in child mortality. *Archs. Dis. Childh.* **45,** 33–38.

Rogers, S. (1970). Skills for genetic engineers. *New Scient.* **45,** 194–196.

Scriver, C. R. (1969). Treatment of inherited disease: realized and potential. *Med. Clins N. Am.* **53**(4), 941–963.

Smith, C. (1970). Ascertaining those at risk in the prevention and treatment of genetic disease. In *Modern Trends in Human Genetics.* Vol. 1. Ed. Emery, A. E. H. pp. 350–369. London: Butterworths.

Smith, C. (1972). Computer program to estimate recurrence risks for multifactorial familial disease. *Brit. med. J.* **1,** 495–497.

Stevenson, A. C. & Davison, B. C. (1970). *Genetic Counselling.* London: Heinemann.

Tips, R. L. and Lynch, H. T. (1963). The impact of genetic counseling upon the family mileu. *J. Am. med. Ass.* **184,** 183–186.

Tips, R. L., Smith, G. S., Lynch, H. T. *et al.* (1964). The 'whole family' concept in clinical genetics. *Am. J. Dis. Child.* **107,** 66–76.

Witkop, C. J., Nance, W. E., Rawis, R. F. *et al.* (1970). Autosomal recessive oculocutaneous albinism in man: evidence for genetic heterogeneity. *Am. J. hum. Genet.* **22,** 55–74.

Glossary

Allele (=allelomorph). Alternative forms of a gene found at the same locus on homologous chromosomes.

Amino acid. An organic compound containing both carboxyl (—COOH) and amino groups (—NH₂).

Anaphase. The stage of cell division when the chromosomes leave the equatorial plate and migrate to opposite poles of the spindle.

Aneuploid. A chromosome number which is not an exact multiple of the haploid number, i.e. $2N-1$ or $2N+1$ where N is the haploid number of chromosomes.

Antibody (=immunoglobulin). A serum protein which is formed in response to an antigenic stimulus and reacts specifically with this antigen.

Anticipation. The *apparent* tendency for some diseases to begin at an earlier age and to increase in severity with each succeeding generation.

Antigen. A substance which elicits the synthesis of antibody with which it also reacts specifically.

Ascertainment. The finding and selection of families with an hereditary disorder.

Association. The occurrence of a particular allele in a group of patients more often than can be accounted for by chance.

Assortative mating (=non-random mating). The preferential selection of a spouse with a particular genotype.

Autosome. Any chromosome other than the sex chromosomes. In man there are 22 pairs of autosomes.

Bacteriophage (=phage). A virus which infects bacteria.

Centromere (=kinetochore). The point at which the two chromatids of a chromosome are joined, and the region of the chromosome which becomes attached to the spindle during cell division.

Chiasma. The cross configuration of chromatids of homologous chromosomes during the first meiotic division.

Chimaera. An individual composed of two populations of cells with different genotypes.

Chromatid. During cell division each chromosome divides longitudinally into two strands of chromatids which are held together by the centromere.

Chromosomal aberration. An abnormality of chromosome number or structure.

Chromosomes. Thread-like, deep staining bodies situated within the nucleus. They are composed of DNA and protein and carry genetic information. An *acrocentric* chromosome is one in which the centromere is located near the end of the chromosome, a *metacentric* chromosome is one in which the centromere is located near the middle of the chromosome.

Cistron. The smallest unit of genetic material which is responsible for the synthesis of a specific polypeptide.

Clone. All the cells derived from a single cell by repeated mitoses and all having the same genetic constitution.

Codominance. When both alleles are expressed in the heterozygote.

Codon. A sequence of three adjacent nucleotides which codes for one amino acid or chain termination.

Concordance. When both members of a pair of twins exhibit the same trait they are said to be concordant. If only one twin has the trait they are said to be discordant.

Congenital. Any abnormality, whether genetic or not, which is present at birth.

Consanguineous marriage. A marriage between ' blood relatives ', that is, between persons who have one or more common ancestors, usually a marriage between first cousins.

Cross-over (=recombination). The exchange of genetic material between chromosomes.

Cytogenetics. A branch of genetics concerned principally with the study of chromosomes.

Cytoplasm. The ground substance of the cell in which are situated the nucleus, endoplasmic reticulum and mitochondria, etc.

Deletion. A type of chromosomal aberration in which there is a loss of a part of a chromosome.

Dermatoglyphics. The patterns of skin ridges on the fingers, toes, palms, and soles.

Diploid. The condition in which the cell contains two sets of chromosomes. Normal state of somatic cells in man, where the diploid number ($2N$) is 46.

Dizygotic (=fraternal). Type of twins produced by the fertilization of two different ova by two different sperms. Dizygotic twins are no more similar genetically than are brothers and sisters.

DNA (=deoxyribonucleic acid). The nucleic acid in chromosomes and in which genetic information is coded.

Dominant. A trait which is expressed in individuals who are heterozygous for a particular gene.

Drift (=random genetic drift). Fluctuations in gene frequencies which tend to occur in small isolated populations.

Duplication. A type of chromosomal aberration in which part of a chromosome is duplicated.

Endoplasmic reticulum. A system of minute tubules within the cytoplasm.

Enzyme. A protein which acts as a catalyst in biological systems.

Expressivity. Variation in severity of the expression of a particular gene.

First-degree relatives. Closest relatives, that is, parents, offspring and sibs.

Fitness (biological fitness). The number of offspring who reach reproductive age. Fitness is unity (or 100 per cent) if he or she has two such offspring.

Gamete. A germ cell (sperm or ovum) containing a haploid number of chromosomes.

Gene. A part of the DNA molecule which directs the synthesis of a specific polypeptide chain. It is composed of many codons. When the gene is considered as a unit of function in this way, the term cistron is often used.

Genotype. The genetic constitution of an individual.

Haploid. The condition in which the cell contains one set of chromosomes. Normal state of gametes in man where the haploid number (N) is 23.

Hemizygous. A term used when describing the genotype of a male with regard to an X-linked trait, since males have only one set of X-linked genes.

Heritability. The proportion of the total variation of a character attributable to genetic as opposed to environmental factors.

Heterogametic sex. The sex which produces gametes of two types. In humans, the male is the heterogametic sex because he produces X- and Y-bearing sperms.

Heterozygote (=carrier). An individual who possesses two different alleles at one particular locus on a pair of homologous chromosomes.

Holandric inheritance. The pattern of inheritance of genes on the Y chromosome: only males are affected and the trait is transmitted by affected males to all their sons but to none of their daughters.

Homogametic sex. The sex which produces gametes of only one type. In humans the female is the homogametic sex bceause she produces only X-bearing ova.

Homograft. Graft between individuals of the same species but with different genotypes.

Homologous chromosomes. Chromosomes which pair during meiosis and contain identical loci.

Homozygote. An individual who possesses two identical alleles at one particular locus on a pair of homologous chromosomes.

Hybrid. The progeny of a cross between two genetically different organisms.

Immunoglobulin. See antibody.

Incompatibility. A donor and host are incompatible if the latter rejects a graft from the former.

Interphase. The stage between two successive cell divisions during which DNA replication occurs.

Inversion. A type of chromosomal aberration in which part of a chromosome is inverted.

Isochromosome. A type of chromosomal aberration in which one of the arms of a particular chromosome is duplicated because the centromere divides transversely and not longitudinally during cell division. The two arms of an isochromosome are therefore of equal length and contain the same genes.

Karyotype. The number, size, and shape of the chromosomes of a somatic cell. A photomicrograph of an individual's chromosomes arranged in a standard manner.

Linkage. Two genes at different loci on the same pair of homologous chromosomes are said to be linked.

Locus. The site of a gene on a chromosome.

Meiosis. The type of cell division which occurs during gametogenesis and results in halving of the somatic number of chromosomes so that each gamete is haploid.

Metaphase. The stage of cell division when the chromosomes line up on the equatorial plate and the nuclear membrane disappears.

Mimic genes. Different genes with similar effects.

Mitochondria. Minute structures situated within the cytoplasm which are concerned with cell respiration.

Mitosis. The type of cell division which occurs in somatic cells.

Monosomy. Loss of one member of a chromosome pair so that there is one less than the diploid number of chromosomes ($2N-1$).

Monozygotic (=identical). Type of twins derived from a single fertilized ovum.

Mosaic. An individual with abnormal genotypic or phenotypic variation from cell to cell within the same tissue or genotypic variation between tissues.

Multifactorial. Inheritance controlled by many genes with small additive effects (polygenic) plus the effects of environment.

Multiple alleles. The existence of more than two alleles at a particular locus in a population.

Mutation (=sport). A change in the genetic material, either of a single gene (point mutation) or in the number or structure of the chromosomes. A mutation which occurs in the gametes is inherited, a mutation which occurs in the somatic cells (somatic mutation) is not inherited.

Mutation rate. The number of mutations of any one particular locus which occur per gamete per generation.

Non-disjunction. The failure of two members of a chromosome pair to disjoin (=separate) during cell division to that both pass to the same daughter cell.

Nucleolus. A structure within the nucleus, the function of which is obscure.

Nucleotide. Nucleic acid is made up of many nucleotides each of which consists of a nitrogenous base, a pentose sugar, and a phosphate group.

Nucleus. A structure within the cell which contains the chromosomes and nucleolus.

Operator gene. A gene which switches on adjacent structural gene(s).

Operon. According to the operon theory an operon is a unit of gene action consisting of an operator gene and the closely linked structural gene(s) which it controls.

Penetrance. When the expression of a genotype is less than 100 per cent then the genotype is said to show reduced penetrance.

Pharmacogenetics. The study of genetically determined variations in drug metabolism.

Phenocopy. A condition which is due to environmental factors but resembles one which is genetic.

Phenotype. The appearance (physical, biochemical, and physiological) of an individual which results from the interaction of environment and his genotype.

Plasmagene. Genes situated within the cytoplasm of the cell.

Pleiotropy. A gene with multiple effects is said to be pleiotropic.

Polymorphism. The occurrence in a population of two or more genetically determined forms in such frequencies that the rarest of them could not be maintained by mutation alone.

Polypeptide. An organic compound consisting of three or more amino acids.

Polyploid. Any multiple of the haploid number of chromosomes (e.g. $3N$, $4N$, etc.).

Polysome (=polyribosome). A group of ribosomes associated with the same molecule of messenger RNA.

Proband (=index case). An affected individual (irrespective of sex) through whom the family came to the attention of the investigator. Propositus if a male; proposita if a female.

Prophase. The first visible stage of cell division when the chromosomes are contracted and therefore thicker.

Protein. A complex organic compound composed of hundreds or thousands of amino acids.

Rad. A measure of the amount of any ionizing radiation which is *absorbed* by the tissues. One rad is equivalent of 100 ergs of energy absorbed per gram of tissue.

Random mating (=panmixis). Selection of a spouse regardless of the spouse's genotype.

Recessive. A trait which is expressed in individuals who are homozygous for a particular gene but not in those who are heterozygous for this gene.

Regulator gene. According to the operon theory a regulator gene synthesizes a repressor substance which inhibits the action of a specific operator gene.

Rem. The dose of any radiation which has the same biological effect as one rad of X-rays.

Ribosomes. Minute spherical structures in the cytoplasm. They are rich in RNA and the seat of protein synthesis.

RNA (=ribonucleic acid). The nucleic acid which is found mainly in the nucleolus and ribosomes. *Messenger-RNA* transfers genetic information from the nucleus to the ribosomes in the cytoplasm and also acts as a template for the synthesis of polypeptides. *Transfer-RNA* transfers activated amino acids from the cytoplasm to messenger-RNA.

Segregation. The separation of alleles during meiosis so that each gamete contains only one member of each pair of alleles.

Selection. The forces which affect biological fitness and therefore the frequency of a particular condition within a given population.

Sex chromatin (=Barr body). A dark-staining mass situated at the periphery of the nucleus during interphase. It represents a single, inactive, condensed X chromosome. The number of sex chromatin masses is one less than the number of X chromosomes (e.g. none in normal males and in XO females, one in normal females and XXY males, etc.).

Sex chromosomes. The chromosomes responsible for sex (XX in women, XY in men).

Sex influence. When a genetic trait is expressed more frequently in one sex than another. In the extreme when only one sex is affected this is called *sex limitation.*

Sex linkage. Genes carried on the sex chromosomes. Since there are very few Mendelizing genes on the Y chromosome the term is often used synonymously for X-linkage.

Sib (=sibling). Brother or sister.

Spindle. A structure responsible for the movement of the chromosomes during cell division.

Telophase. The stage of cell division when the chromosomes have completely separated into two groups and each group has become invested in a nuclear membrane.

Teratogen. An agent believed to cause congenital abnormalities.

Transcription. The process whereby genetic information is transmitted from the DNA in the chromosomes to messenger-RNA.

Transformation. The transfer of genetic information to one strain of bacteria by DNA extracted from another strain.

Translation. The process whereby genetic information from messenger-RNA is translated into protein synthesis.

Translocation. The transfer of genetic material from one chromosome to another non-homologous chromosome. If there is an *exchange* of genetic material between two chromosomes then this is referred to as a *reciprocal translocation.*

Triplet. A series of three bases in the DNA or RNA molecule which codes for a specific amino acid.

Triploid. A cell with three times the haploid number of chromosomes (i.e. 3N).

Trisomy. A chromosome additional to the normal complement (i.e. 2N+1) so that in each nucleus one particular chromosome is represented three times rather than twice.

Unifactorial (=Mendelizing). Inheritance controlled by a single gene pair.

X-linkage. Genes carried on the X chromosome are said to be X-linked.

Zygote. The fertilized ovum.

Index

Index

Aberration, chromosome, 10, 60, 205
Abnormalities, congenital, see Congenital abnormalities
ABO blood groups, 10
  association, 126-128, 167
  Bombay types, 23
  codominance, 104
  disputed paternity, 208
  gene frequencies, 160
  linkage, 52
  multiple alleles, 110
  in North American Indians, 160
  random mating and, 157
  and recurrent abortion, 207
Abortion:
  recurrent, 207
  selective, 214
  spontaneous, 206
Abrahamson, S., 185
Acatalasia, 143
  detection of carriers, 209
Achondroplasia, 98
  mutation rate, 154, 155, 156
  reduced reproductive fitness, 155
Acrocentric chromosomes, 45
Adenine, 15
Adenylate kinase, linkage, 54
Adoption, 207
Adrenogenital syndrome, 76, 217
Adult haemoglobin, 32
Agammaglobulinaemia,
  Bruton type, 41
  Swiss type, 41
Age effect, maternal:
  in Down's syndrome, 63, 64
  in Klinefelter's syndrome, 70
  paternal: on sex ratio, 188
Age effect, on mutation rate, 157
Aird, I., 135
Alberman, E., 64
Albinism, 2, 30, 164
  inheritance, 103
  metabolic block, 28, 30
  mutation rate, 156
  ocular, 87, 210, 212
  tyrosinase +ve and −ve, 203

Alkaptonuria, 9
  frequency in population, 153
  inheritance, 103
  metabolic block, 9, 28, 30
Alleles, 5, 223
Allelic system, see Multiple alleles
Allison, A. C., Fig. 42: 168
Am proteins, 39
Amber, 20
Amino acids, 17, 223
  in haemoglobins, 32-37
  in histones, 91
  protein synthesis, 17-22
Amish, 157, 160, 161
Amniotic fluid, 214
Amniocentesis, 214, 215
Amyotrophic lateral sclerosis, 161
Anaemia, sickle-cell, 32
Anaphase, 223
  in meiosis, 48, 49
  in mitosis, 48
Anencephaly, 130
Aneuploidy, 61, 223
  and genetic counselling, 201
  of sex chromosomes, 70
Angiokeratoma (Fabry's disease), 53
Angioneurotic oedema, 29, 217
Angiosarcoma, 132
Anhidrotic ectodermal dysplasia, 87
Animal analogues, 135, 136
Ankylosing spondylitis, 111, 115, 118
Antenatal diagnosis, 214
Antenatal treatment, in mice, 219
  potential in man, 219
Antibodies, 38, 223
Anticipation, in autosomal dominant traits, 195, 223
Anticoagulants, 145
Antigen, 223
Anti-mongolism, 68
Apert's syndrome, 157
Apnoea, 144
Apostatic selection, 169
Argininaemia, 216
Aristotle, 1

Artificial insemination by donor (A.I.D.), 214
Artificial selection, *see* Selection
Aryl hydrocarbon hydroxylase (AHH), 137
Asbestos, 132
Ascertainment, 223
Association, 126, 223
Assortative mating, 157, 223
Ataxia telangiectasia, 41, 133
Atherosclerosis, 125
Atomic bomb, *see* Radiation
Atomic fallout, *see* Radiation
Autoradiography, 58
Autosomal chromosomes, 46, 223
    abnormalities of, 61, 67. *See also* Chromosomes
Autosomal linkage, 51, 211
Autosomal marker traits, 51
Avery, O. T., 13

Bacteriophage, 14, 223
    temperate, 136
Baldness, presenile, 100
Bands in chromosomes, 7. *See also* Puffs
Barr body, 73. *See also* Sex chromatin body
Basal cell nevus syndrome, 133
Bateson, W., 9
Beadle, G. W., 27
Becker, muscular dystrophy, 110, 215
    carrier detection, 212
Beta-amino-isobutyric acid excretion, 172
Biston betularia, 169, 170
Bittner, J. J., 135, 136
Blindness:
    in man, 103; in mice, 219
Blood groups:
    Duffy, 52, 211
    Lutheran, 52
    MNS, 54
    Rhesus, 52
    Xg, 52, 109. *See also* ABO
Bloom's syndrome, 133
Bombay blood group, 23. *See also* ABO blood groups
Borden, E. C., 136
Boveri, T., 6
Brachydactyly, 99
Bridges, C. B., 51, 63
Briggs, R., 83

Britten-Davidson model, 25
Bruton's agammaglobulinaemia, 37, 133
Bullough, W. S., 92

Cancer, 131
    animal studies, 135
    and chromosomes, 61
    family and twin studies, 134
    inheritance, 117
    of breast, 117, 134, 135
    of cervix, 132
    of eye, 132
    of large intestine, 132
    of nervous system, 132
    of penis, 132
    of skin, 132
    of stomach, 134
        association with blood groups, 135
Candela, P. B., 161
Carr, D. H., 206
Carriers:
    of acatalasia, 209
    of autosomal recessive disorders, 197
    of Crigler-Najjar syndrome, 148
    of Down's syndrome, 64, 65, 66
    of Duchenne muscular dystrophy, 108, 212
    of galactosaemia, 210
    of haemophilia, 50, 107, 210
    recognition, 209
    selection against, 165
    in X-linked disorders, 212
Carter, C. O., 114, 130, 213
Cartilage-hair hypoplasia syndrome, 158
Casey, M. D., 72
Castle, W. E., 6
Catalase, deficiency of, 142, 143
Cataract, 28, 30
    linkage, 52, 211
Cattle twins, 78
Cell, animal, 12
    hybridization, 52, 53
Centromere, 45, 223
    and isochromosomes, 79
Chalones, 92
Chase, M., 14
Chediak-Higashi syndrome, 133
Chiasma, 223
Chimaera, 77, 223

Chlorothiazide, 147
Chordamesoderm, 88
Chromatid, 47, 223
Chromatin, sex, 73, 87
Chromosome, 6, 12, 224
  aberration, 223
  incidence at birth, 77
  in abortions, spontaneous, 206
  autosomal, 46, 51, 61
  banding methods, 59
  and cancer, 61
  deletions, 64, 66, 79, 224
  and disease, 61, 69, 70
  duplications, 225
  fluorescence, 59, 60, 73, 74
  and genetic counselling, 205
  heteropyknotic, 87
  homologous, 45, 48, 49, 50
  identification, 58
  inversion, 79
  isochromosome, 79
  and leukaemia, 69
  non-disjunction, 63, 119
  number, 10, 46, 56
  Philadelphia, 69
  ring, 66, 79
  salivary gland of Drosophila, 7, 85
  sex, 46
    abnormalities of, 10, 70, 79, 205
  shorthand, 68
  technique of growing, 56
  translocations, 64-66, 206, 229. See
    also Autosome, X chromo-
    some and Y chromosome
Chronic granulomatous disease, 212
Cistron, 37, 224
Clarke, C. A., 220
Cleft hand, 202
Cleft lip and palate, 130
  empiric risk, 210
Clone, 224
Club foot, 130
Code, genetic, 17
  degenerate, 20
  mutation and, 22
Codominance, 104, 224
Codon, 17, 224
Coefficient of selection against the
  gene, 155, 163
Colchicine in tissue culture, 56
Colour blindness, 52, 105, 166
  partial, 107
  polymorphism, 172

Concordant twins, 119, 224. See also
  Twins
Congenital abnormalities, 130, 224
  environmental factors, 90, 200, 202
  genetic counselling, 200-201, 202.
    See also specific malforma-
    tions
Congenital cataract, linkage, 52, 53,
  54
Congenital dislocation of the hip, 130
  in dogs, 135
  empiric risks, 210
  heritability, 115
Congenital heart disease, 130
  and rubella, 202-203
Congestive heart failure, 147
Conjugation, glucuronide, 140
  of bilirubin, 148
  deficiency of glucuronyl trans-
    ferase, 148
  carrier detection, 148
Consanguinity, 7, 10, 224
  in autosomal recessive inheritance,
    102, 103, 204. See also In-
    breeding, Cousin marriages
Control gene, see Gene control
Cornea, in the mucopolysaccharid-
  oses, 199
Corona radiata, 83
Coronary artery disease, see Ischae-
  mic heart disease
Correns, C., 6
Cosmic rays, 178
Coumarin, 145
Counselling, see Genetic counselling
Cousin marriages, 7, 8, 204, 224
  frequency of, 103. See also In-
    breeding
  genetic counselling, 197, 204, 205
Cowie, V., 130
Creasy, M. R., 62
Creatine kinase, 211
Cretinism, Fig. 6: 28, 217
Crick, F. H. C., 15
Cri du chat syndrome, 66, 67
  genetic counselling in, 201
Crigler-Najjar syndrome, 148
Crolla, J. A., 62
Crossing over, 50-51, 224
  between sex chromosomes, 104-105
Cultural selection, albinism, 161
Culture, tissue, 56-58
Curare, 144

Cystathioninuria, 216
Cystinuria, 30, 164
Cytogenetics, 56, 224. *See also*
Chromosomes
Cytoplasm, 12, 224
Cytoplasmic inheritance, *see* Extra-
chromosomal inheritance
Cytosine, 15

Damon, A., 158
Darlington, C. D., 80
Darwin, C., 5, 7, 8
Davenport, C. B., 9
DDT resistance, 139
Deafness, 8, 103
caused by rubella, 203
profound childhood, 210
Deletions, of a gene, 37. *See also*
Chromosomes
Denborough, M. A., 146
Deoxyribonucleic acid (DNA), 15,
224
in chromosomes, 16
genetic code and, 17
replication, 17
structure, 15-17
transcription, 19
transformation, 13-14
translation, 19
Dermatoglyphics, 74, 224
ridge count, 111
De Grouchy, J., 67, 68
De Vries, H., 6
Diabetes insipidus, nephrogenic, 90,
212
Diabetes mellitus, 118
congenital abnormalities in infants
of mothers with, 118, 119, 202
genetic predisposition to, 121
inheritance of, 119-121
twin studies in, 119
Diaphyseal aclasis, 133
Dibucaine number, 144
Di George syndrome, Fig. 9 : 37, 40
Dintzis, H., 20
Diploid, 45, 224
Discordant twins, 119. *See also*
Twins
Disputed paternity, 207
Distribution, normal, 112
Diuretics, 147
Dizygotic, 224
Doll, R., 125

Dominance, arbitrary nature of, 2,
104
Dominant, 3, 224
Dominant inheritance, 3, 97
autosomal, 97, 200
sex-linked, 109. *See also* Intermediate inheritance.
Dosage compensation, 87
Down's syndrome, 10, 61, 67, 117
dermal ridge patterns in, 75
genetic counselling, 63, 64, 201,
207
leukaemia and, 62
mosaicism and, 77
non-disjunction and, 63
Dreyfus, J. C., 25
Drift, *see* Random genetic drift
Drosophila melanogaster, 6, 7
chromosome map, 51
effect of X-rays on, 182
genetic load in, 187
lethal mutants in, 90, 187
salivary gland chromosomes, 7
somatic mutations in, 184
Drug, metabolism of, 139-141
conjugation, 140
genetic variability, 141-146
response in hereditary disorders,
146-149
therapy, cholestyramine, penicillamine, phenobarbitone, 218
Drug, effects of, in pregnancy, 202.
See also Pharmacogenetics
Drumsticks, 73, 74
Duchenne, G. B. A., 108
Duchenne muscular dystrophy, 107
Duffy blood group, 52
linkage, 53, 54, 211
Dunkers, 161
Duodenal ulcer, 125, 126, 127
association with blood group O,
126
Duplications, 225. *See also* Chromo-
somes
Dwarfs:
sexual ateliotic, 90
Dysgammaglobulinaemias, 41

Ears, hairy, 75, 110
Ecdysone, 85, 89
Edwards, J. H., 115
Edward's syndrome, 62, 67
Eicher, E. M., 207

Electrophoresis, 93, 171. *See also*
Isozymes, Serum proteins
Elliptocytosis, 52, 54
Ellis-van Creveld syndrome, 160, 161
Embryonic haemoglobin, 32
Embryonic induction, 88
Emery, A. E. H., 214, 219
Empiric risk, 193, 209, 210
Endoplasmic reticulum, 12, 225
Environment and heredity, 9, 114, 117
Enzymes, 10, 225
in detection of carriers, 211
gene control of, 23
as gene products, 27
in metabolic blocks, 27-31. *See also* Isozymes
Epilepsy, 162, 210
Epiloia, 133
mutation rate, 156
Escherichia coli, 23
Eugenics, 8, 162-164, 174. *See also* Genetic counselling
Evans, D. A. P., 146
Evolution, 5
non-Darwinian, 173
Expressivity, 99, 202, 225
Extrachromosomal inheritance, 80

Fabry's disease, carrier detection, 212. *See also* Angiokeratoma
Falconer, D. S., 115
Fallout, *see* Radiation
Fanconi's anaemia, 133
Farabee, W. C., 99
Favism, 145
Ferguson-Smith, M. A., 76
Fertility and intelligence, 174
Fertilization, in animals, 82
double, 77
in man, 82-83
multiple, 83
Fetal haemoglobin, 32
Fibrocystic disease, 102, 164, 213
Filial, 2
First-degree relatives, 225
Fisher, R. A., 5, 111, 166
Fitness, 162, 225
Follicles, ovarian, *see* Graafian follicles
Ford, C. E., 10, 70, 73
Ford, E. B., 167
Forme fruste, 195

Founder effect, 158
Freemartins, 78
Frequency, distribution curve, 112
Friedmann, T., 218
Frog embryology, experimental, 84

G chromosome translocation, 64-66
genetic counselling and, 66, 207
Galactose, 28
Galactosaemia, 27, 28
metabolic block, 28
Galton, F., 8
Gamete, 4, 45, 225
and meiosis, 48
Gametogenesis, 50, 72
Gammaglobulins, *see* Immunoglobulins
Gardner, R. J. M., 156
Gargoylism, Hunter's syndrome, 199, 201
carrier detection in, 212
treatment of, 217
Hurler's syndrome, 199
Garrod, A. E., 9, 27
Gastric ulcer, 125, 126, 127
Gaussian distribution, 112
Gc serum proteins:
linkage, 54
Gene, 5, 6, 7, 35, 225
action, 17, 32
artificial, 22
control (modifier), 23
Britten-Davidson model, 25, 26
Jacob and Monod's model, 25
control of enzymes, 10, 23
control by histones, 91
control by hormones, 85, 86, 89-90, 92-93
cytoplasmic, 80
derepression, 85
enzyme synthesis and, 10, 27
extinguished, 159
fixed, 159
flow, 161
frequency in population, 151
inducer, 25
lethal mutant, 90
linked, 51
mimic, 203
marker, 51
mutant, 20, 29, 35, 50
neutral, 166
operator, 24

Gene—*continued*
  penetrant, incompletely, 111
  non-, 100, 195
  pleiotropic, 35
  polypeptide synthesis and, 37
  recombination, 50
  regulator, 24
  repression, 24, 84, 88, 91
  structural, 22
  super-repressor, 25
  synthesis of, 22
Genetic code, 17-22
  mutation and, 20
Genetic counselling, 8, 9, 191, 194
  acceptability of genetic risks, 213
  autosomal dominant traits, 194
  anticipation in, 195
  autosomal recessive traits, 196
  chromosome studies, 205
  cousin marriages, 7, 197, 204
  empiric risk, 209
  familial incidence and, 115
  infertility and, 206
  problems in, 201-204
  sporadic case, 199
  X-linked recessive traits, 197-199
Genetic drift, *see* Random genetic
    drift
Genetic engineering, 218
Genetic heterogeneity, 203
Genetic load, 171, 187
Genetic predisposition to disease, 219
  recognition of preclinical cases, 219
Genetic register, 219
Genotype, 8, 225
Giemsa staining, 59
Glass, B., 1
Glaucoma, 148
Globulin, antihaemophilic, 29, 87
  Ig, 38
Glucose-6-phosphate dehydrogenase
    deficiency, 52, 107, 145, 149
  carriers, 212
  selective advantage, 170
  X-linkage, 107
Glucuronide conjugation, 140, 148
Glucuronyl transferase, deficiency of,
    148
  induction of, 218
Glutamic acid in Hb, 33
Gm proteins, 51
Gout, 100, 147
Graafian follicles, 1

Griffith, F., 13
Guanine, 15
Gurdon, J. B., 83
Guthrie test, 28

Haemoglobin, structure of, 32
Haemoglobin A, 32
Haemoglobin C, 35
Haemoglobin Chesapeake, 36
Haemoglobin Constant Spring, 37
Haemoglobin F (Hull), 36
Haemoglobin Flatbush, 36
Haemoglobin Heathrow, 36
Haemoglobin J (Capetown), 36
Haemoglobin Kansas, 36
Haemoglobin M (Boston), 36
Haemoglobin S, 33, 34, 35, 36, 104
  codominance, 104
  selective advantage, 167-169, 170
Haemoglobin Tak, 37
Haemoglobin Zurich, 36, 147
Haemoglobinopathies, 32-38
  drug response in, 147
Haemophilia A, 1
  carriers of, 212
  cause, 29
  in dogs, 135
  mutation rate, 156
  sex-linkage, 7, 53, 105
Haemophilia B:
  carriers of, 212
Hairy ears, 75, 110
Halothane, in malignant hyper-
    pyrexia, 146
Hamerton, J. L., 10
Haploid, 45, 225
Haptoglobins, 171
Hardy, G. H., 151
Hardy-Weinberg principle, 151
  factors affecting, 154
  effect of inbreeding, 157
  mutation, 154
  random genetic drift, 158
  selection, 162
Harris, H., 173
Harvey, W., 1
Hemizygous, 105, 225
Henking, H., 46
Heredity and environment, 9, 114,
    117
Heritability, 114, 225
  in diabetes mellitus, 121
  in ischaemic heart disease, 125

Heritability—*continued*
 in peptic ulcer, 128
 in schizophrenia, 130
Hermaphroditism, 75
Herndon, C. N., 209
Hershey, A. D., 14
Heston, L. L., 128
Heterogametic sex, 225
Heterosis, 167. *See also* Polymorphism, genetic
Heterozygote, 4, 225
 manifesting, 108
 selective advantage in, 167
Heuch, I., 194
Hippocrates, 100
Hirschsprung's disease, 210
Histocompatibility locus-A, 42
Histones, 91
 and gene control, 91-92
Holandric inheritance, 110, 225. *See also* Y-linked inheritance
Homocystinuria, 217
Homogametic sex, 225
Homogentisic acid in alkaptonuria, 9, 28
Homologous chromosomes, 45, 48, 49, 50, 225
Homozygote, 4, 226
 in autosomal dominant inheritance, 97
 in autosomal recessive inheritance, 100
Hook, E. B., 72
Hormones, 85, 89, 92
Hunter's syndrome, 199
Huntington's chorea, 193, 195
Hurler's syndrome, 199
Hybrid, 3, 52, 53, 226
Hybrid vigor, 167. *See also* Poylmorphism, genetic
Hydralazine, 144
Hydrocephalus, congenital, 207
Hydrogen bonds in DNA, 15
Hydrogen peroxide, 141-143
Hydrometrocolpos, 158
Hypercholesterolaemia, 29, 125, 218.
Hyperpyrexia, 146
Hypertension, 122
Hypogammaglobulinaemias, 41
Hypoproteinaemia, 216

Ichthyosis vulgaris, X-linked, 53
Iduronosulphate sulphatase, 30

Immunoglobulins, 38-42, 226
 Fab fragment, 38
 Fc fragment, 38
Inactivation of X chromosome, 86-88
Inborn error of metabolism, 10, 27
Inbreeding, 7, 8, 157
Incest, 205
Incompatibility, 226
Incomplete dominance, 104
Induction, embryonic, *see* Embryonic induction
 enzymic, 217, 218
Infertility and genetic counselling, 206
Ingram, V. M., 33
Inheritance, multifactorial, 111, 191-193
 simple, 193
Insect larvae, development of, 85
Intelligence, 111
 multifactorial inheritance of, 111, 112
Intelligence and fertility, 174
Intermediate inheritance, 103-104
Interphase, 47, 226
Inv proteins, 41
Inversion, 79, 226
Ionizing radiations, 177-178
 artificial, 179-181
 natural, 178-179
Ir locus, 43
Ischaemic heart disease, 125
Isochromosome, 79, 226
Isoenzyme, *see* Isozyme
Isolates, genetic, 157, 158
Isoniazid, 141, 143
 inactivation, 140
 rapid, 143
 slow, 143
 treatment of tuberculosis with, 143
Isozyme, 93

Jacob, F., 23, 25
Jacobs, P. A., 10, 70
Johannsen, W., 5, 8
Johnstone, E. C., 144
Jost, A., 75

Käosaar, M. E., 207
Karyotype, 58, 226
Khorana, H. G., 22
Kinetochore, *see* Centromere, 223
King, T. J., 83

Klinefelter's syndrome, 70
  mosaicism in, 77
Knight, T. A., 2
Koulischer, L., 80

Lactate dehyrogenase (LDH), 93
Landsteiner, K., 10
Leber's optic atrophy, 80
Lejeune, J., 10, 61, 66
Lesch-Nyhan syndrome, 30-31, 53, 212
Lethal mutant, 90
Leucocytes, see Drumsticks
Leukaemia, 61, 69
  chronic granulocytic, 69
  in mice, 135
  mongolism and, 62
  and radiation, 182
Levan, A., 10, 56, 61
Li, F. H. F., 194
Liability to develop disease, 112
Linkage, genetic, 50, 226
  autosomal vs. association, 126
  in carrier recognition, 211
  X chromosome, 104-110
  Y chromosome, 75, 104, 110
  maps, 51
  studies in man, 51, 52, 53, 54, 55. See also Sex linkage
Lobster claw, 202
Locus, chromosomal, 226
Lucké, kidney cancer in frogs, 136
Lutheran blood groups, 52, 54
Lyon hypothesis, 86
Lyon, M. F., 86
Lyonization, 86, 108
Lysine in Hb C, 35

McArdle's syndrome, 31
McCarty, M., 13
Macklin, M. T., 134
McKusick's syndrome, 158
MacLeod, C. M., 13
Malaria, falciparum, 169, 170
Malignant hyperpyrexia, 146
Manifesting heterozygote, 108
Map, chromosome 51. See also Recombination
Map units, 51
Maple syrup urine, 30-31, 217
Marfan's syndrome, 208
Marker genes, 51
Marsh, W., 144
Maternal age effect, 63-64, 70, 157

Maternal inheritance, see Extrachromosomal inheritance
Matthaei, J. H., 19
Maupertuis, P. L. M., 1, 2, 7
McDougall, J. K., 60
Meiosis, 48-50, 226. See also Nondisjunction
Meiotic studies in humans, 79
Melanin, 28
  in skin cancer, 132
Mendel, G., 2, 3, 5
Mendelian inheritance, chromosomes and, 50
Mendelism, 2-6
Ménière, P., 8
Mental retardation:
  and sex chromosomes, 72
  inheritance, 9
  empiric risk, 201, 210
Merril, C. R., 218
Metabolic block, 27-32
Metabolism, inborn error of, 10, 30-31
Metacentric chromosomes, 45
Metaphase, 226
  in meiosis, 48, 49
  in mitosis, 47
Methaemoglobinaemia, 36
Methylmalonic-acidaemia, 216
Mice, cancer in, 135
  dwarf mutant, 89
  eye defect, 219
  hare lip, 219
  leukaemia, 69, 135
  pygmy mutant, 89
Microcephaly, 202
Miescher, F., 13, 91
Mikelsaar, A-V. N., 207
Milk, agent, 136
Mimic genes, 203, 226
Mitochondria, 13, 226
Mitosis, 47, 226
Mixed lymphocyte culture, 42
MNS blood group, linkage, 54, 55
Mongolism, see Down's syndrome
Monod, J., 23, 25
Monosomy, 61, 226
  partial, 66
Monozygotic, 226
Moulds, R. F. W., 146
Mørch, T. E., 155
Morgan, T. H., 51
Morris, J. N., 123

Morrison, S. L., 123
Morton, N. E., 111
Mosaicism, 76, 77, 226
  gonadic, 202
  in hermaphrodites, 76
Mucoviscidosis, see Fibrocystic disease
Muller, H. J., 182
Multifactorial inheritance, 9, 111, 226. See also Heritability
  in diabetes, 121
  in drug metabolism, 141
  in hypertension, 122
  familial incidence, 111, 114, 115
  liability to develop disease, 112
  population incidence, 113
  threshold, 112
Multigenic inheritance, see Multifactorial inheritance
Multiple allele, 41, 110, 226
Muscular dystrophy:
  allelic system in, 110
  Becker type, 110, 215
  detection of carriers of, 198, 211, 212
  Duchenne type, 51, 107, 108, 110, 165, 198, 201, 203
  facio-scapulo-humeral type, 203
  limb-girdle type, 203
  in mice, 135
  mutation rate, 156
Mutagens, chemical, 186, 187
Mutant gene, see Gene, mutant
Mutation, 98, 154, 226-227
  cause, 182-183, 186
  base substitution, 20
  chromosome, 182-183
  lethal, see Lethal mutant
  point, 182
  radiation-induced, 182, 183, 184
  rate, 227
    doubling of, 186
  measurement of, direct method, 154
    indirect method, 155
  selection and, 162
  somatic, 184
  spontaneous, 184, 186
  temperature and, 187
  termination, 37
Myotonic dystrophy, 196
  immunoglobulins in, 42
Myxoma in rabbits, 136

Nägeli, C., 6
Nail-patella syndrome, 52
  linkage, 126
Nance, W. E., 131
Nasse's law, 107
Natural selection, 162. See also Population genetics
Nature vs. nurture, 8
Neel, J. V., 187, 188
Negroes, blood group genes, 162
  red cell G6PD deficiency, 145
Neoplasm, 131
Neurofibromatosis, 133
Neurospora crassa, 10, 51
Nevin, N. C., 125
Nirenberg, M. W., 19
Non-disjunction, 63, 64, 72, 77, 227
  secondary, 63
Normal distribution, 112
North American Indians, 160, 161
Nucleic acid, and genetic information, 13-16
  transformation, 13-14. See also Deoxyribonucleic acid, Ribonucleic acid
Nucleotide structure, 15, 227
Nucleolus, Fig. 1: 12, 15, 227
Nucleo-protein in embryonic induction, 88, 89
Nucleus, 6, Fig. 1: 12, 83, 84, 227

Ochre, 20
Ocular, albinism, 53, 87, 212
Oncogenic viruses, 136
Operator gene, 24, 227
Operon, 24, 227
Oroticaciduria, 25
Osteogenesis imperfecta, 96, 98, 110
  expressivity, 99
Outbreeding, 8
Ova, 82-83

Painter, T. S., 56
Panamixis, 157, 228
Paris nomenclature, 60
Parsons, P. A., 171
Partial sex linkage, 104
Patau, K., 62, 67
Paternal age, effect, 157
Pauling, L., 33
PEDIG, 194
Pedigree:
  in diagnosis, 96

Pedigree—*continued*
  showing patterns of inheritance,
    96, 108
Pendred's syndrome, 220
Penetrance, 195, 227
Penicillin resistance, 139
Peppered moth, 164, 169, 170
Peptic ulcer, 117, 125
  concordance in twins, 125, 126
  heritability, 128
Peroneal muscular atrophy, 203
Peyer's patches, 38
Phaeochromocytoma, 133
Pharmacogenetics, 139-150, 227
Phaseolus vulgaris, 56
Phenelzine, 144
Phenocopy, 227
  in genetic counselling, 202
Phenocritical period, 90
Phenotype, 8, 227
Phenylalanine, 20
  causing fetal brain damage, 204
Phenylalanine hydroxylase, 27
Phenylalaninaemia, 28
Phenylbutazone, 146
Phenylketonuria, 27, 204, 217, 219
  in cousin marriages, 204, 205
  genetic counselling, 204
  metabolic block, 27
  in monkeys, 135
  mutation rate, 156
Phenylpyruvic acid, in
  phenylketonuria, 27
Phenylthiocarbamide, *see* PTC
  tasting
Philadelphia chromosome, 69
Phosphoglycerate kinase, 53
Phytohaemagglutinin, 56
Pisum sativum, 2-6
Pituitary gland of mice, 89
Plasmagene, 80, 227. *See also* Extra-
  chromosomal inheritance
Plasmapheresis, 220. *See also* Rh
  incompatibility
Platt, R., 122, 124
Pleiotropy, 35, 227
Pneumococcus, transformation of, 13
Polycystic kidney disease, adult type,
  208
Polydactyly, 2, 5, 10, 32
  expressivity, 99
Polygenic inheritance, *see* Multifac-
  torial inheritance

Polymorphism,   genetic,   167-173,
    227
  balanced, 167
  cytogenic, 59
  geographic, 167-171, 172
  in sickle cell anaemia, 168
  transient, 167, 169
Polypeptides, 227
  gene control of, 37
Polyploidy, 61, 227
Polyposis coli, 132, 133, 219
  mutation rate, 156
Polysome, 19, 227
Polyvinyl chloride (P.V.C.), 132
Population genetics, 151-174
Porphyria acute intermittent, 29
  erythropoetic, 25
  variegata, 98, 147
Prediabetics, 121, 219
Primaquine sensitivity, 145
Probability, 193
  calculation of, 193-194, 198
  conditional, 193, 198
  joint, 193, 198
  posterior or relative, 193, 198
  prior, 193, 198
Proband, 227
Progestins, synthetic, 90
Prophase, 228
  in meiosis, 48
  in mitosis, 47
Propionic-acidaemia, 216
Proposita, 96
Propositus, 96
Proteins, 17, 228
  genes and, 27-32
  genetic code and, 17-22
  serum, 171-173
  synthesis,
    control of, 22, 84, 85
    in vitro, 19, 20
    in vivo, 23, 24. *See also* Immuno-
      globulins, Haemoglobin
Pseudocholinesterase, 144-145, 149
PTC tasting, 51, 166, 172
  polymorphism, 172
  and thyroid disease, 166
Puffs, 85
Punnett, R. C., 4
Purines in nucleic acids, 15
Pyloric stenosis, 113-114
  empiric risk, 210
Pyrimidines, in nucleic acids, 15

Quinacrine fluorescence, 59

Racial differences in cancer, 132. *See also* Polymorphisms, genetic
Rad, 177, 228
Radiation, 177-189
  atomic, 177, 179-180, 187
  cosmic, 178
  dose, 177, 184
  during pregnancy, 90, 182, 200, 202
  effects of, 181
  external, 179
  internal, 179
  ionizing, 177
  occupational, 181
  maximum permissible dose, 189
  in medical practice, 180
  sources of, 178

Random genetic drift, 158, 224
  influence on human blood groups, 160
Random mating, *see* Panmixis
RAPID register, 219
Recessive inheritance, 3, 97, 200, 228
  autosomal, 100-103
  sex-linked, 104-110, 201
Recessiveness, arbitrary nature of, 104
von Recklinghausen's disease, 132, 133. *See also* Neurofibromatosis
Recombination, 50
  measurement, 51
Regression coefficient, 8
Regulator gene, 24, 228
Rem, 177, 228
Repression-derepression mechanisms, 84-85, 92-93. *See also* X chromosome inactivation, Gene repression
Resistance to drugs, 139, 145
Response to drugs,
  abnormal, 148
  continuous, 141
  discontinuous, 141
Reticular dysgenesis, 40
Retinoblastoma, 132, 133
Retinoschisis, 53
Retinitis pigmentosa, 212

Rhesus (Rh) blood groups, 52, 54
  incompatibility, 220
  and malaria, 171
  multiple alleles in, 110
  plasmapheresis to remove Rh antibodies, 220
Ribonucleic acid (RNA), 15, 228
  messenger, 17, 18, 19, 20
  protein synthesis and, 17-19
  soluble, 19
  synthesis (DNA-dependent), 91
  template, 18, 19, 20, 22
  transfer, 19, 20
Ribosomes, 13, 228
  in protein synthesis, 18, 19
Rickets, vitamin-D resistant, 109, 212
Ring chromosome, 66
Roblin, R., 218
Rous sarcoma in fowls, 136
Rubella, maternal infection with, 90 202, 203
Ruddle, F. H., 53

Salivary gland chromosomes, 7, 85. *See also* Puffs
Schizoid, 128
Schizophrenia, 128, 219
  empiric risk, 210
Schoysman, R., 80
Schull, W. J., 187
Schwartz, E., 35
Sclerosteosis, 160
Scott, J. S., 76
Secretor locus, 52
  and peptic ulcer, 127, 128
Segregation, 4, 228
Selection, 162, 228
  apostatic, 169
  artificial, 162
  coefficient of, 155, 163
  effect on fitness, 162
  natural, 162
Selective abortion, 214
Serum proteins, 38, 171
  polymorphisms, 171-173
Sex chromatin body, 73-74, 228
  studies of, 215
Sex chromosomes, 46, 228
  abnormalities, 70-77
  mental retardation and, 72
  mosaicism, 76, 77
  structural abnormalities, 79
Sex determination, 46

Sex influence, 100, 228
 in autosomal dominant inheritance,
  100
Sex limitation, *see* Sex influence
Sex linkage, 7, 51, 104-110, 228
 partial, 104
 and selection, 165. *See also* X-
  chromosome linkage
Sex ratio, 188
Shope papilloma in rabbits, 136, 218
Sib, 96, 229
Sibship, 101
Sickle-cell anaemia, 32-35, 104, 164
 polymorphism in, 167-169. *See
  also* Haemoglobin S
Sickle-cell trait, 35, 104, 167-169
Simpson, N. E., 121
Skin colour, 111
Skin grafting, in chimaeras, 78
Slater, E., 130
Smith, C., 115, 121, 209
Smithies, O., 171
Soluble RNA, 19
Spermatogenesis, 48, 49
Spina bifida, 130, 131
Spindle, 47, 56, 229
Sporadic, 196
Stature, 111
Steinberg, A. G., 120
Strong, J. A., 70
Sturtevant, A. H., 7
Succinylcholine, 144, 146
Sucrose intolerance, 25
Sulphasalazine, 144
Superoxide dismutase, 53
Sutton, W. S., 6
Suxamethonium, *see* Succinylcholine
Syndactyly, 213
Syndrome, 62

Takahara, S., 142
Tarkowski, A. K., 78
Tatum, E. L., 10, 27
Taussig, L. M., 102
Tay-Sachs disease, 31
Telophase, 229
 in meiosis, 48
 in mitosis, 48
Temin, H. M., 22
Temperature, effect on mutation
 rate, 187
Template RNA, 18, 19, 20, 22
Teratogenic agent, 90, 200, 229

Testicular feminization syndrome,
 75, 100, 162
Thalassaemia, 37, 169, 170, 212, 213
Thalidomide, 90, 202
Threshold, 112
Thymine, 15
Tissue culture, 56-58
Tissue grafts, 41, 42
Tjio, J. H., 10, 56, 61
Tobacco mosaic virus, 18
Transcription, 19, 229
Transfer RNA, 19
Transferrins, 51, 54, 171
Transformation in bacteria, 13-14,
 229
Translation, 19, 229
Translocation, *see* Chromosomes
Transplantation genetics, 42
 HL-A antigen, 42
 matching, 42
 tissue-typing, 42, 43
Treatment, of genetic diseases, 216
 in utero, 219, 220
Triplet (in genetic code), 17, 19, 20,
 21, 229. *See also* Codon
Triploid, 61, 229
Trisomy, 61, 229
 double, 73
 partial, 66, 68
Trisomy-4p, 67
Trisomy-8 syndrome, 67
Trisomy-9, 67,
Trisomy-10, 70
Trisomy-13 syndrome, 62, 67, 75
 genetic counselling and, 201. *See
  also* Trisomy, partial
Trisomy-18 syndrome, 62, 67, 75
 genetic counselling and, 201
Trisomy-21 syndrome, 62, 67, 75. *See
  also* Down's syndrome
Trisomy-22 syndrome, 67
Trypsinogen deficiency, 216
von Tschermak-Seysenegg, E., 6
Tuberculosis, pulmonary, 117
Turner's syndrome, 70, 108
 genetic counselling, 205, 206
 isochromosomes in, 79
 mosaicism in, 77
 sex chromatin in, 74
Twins, 8, 63
 cancer in, 135
 chimaerism in, 78
 congenital abnormalities, 131

Twins—*continued*
    diabetes mellitus in, 119, 120
    genetic studies and, 118
    heritability and, 115
    identical, 63
    peptic ulcers in 125-126
    schizophrenia, 129
    spina bifida, 131
Tylosis, 133
    linkage, 54
Tyrosinase, 28
Tyrosine, 28

Unifactorial, 229
Uracil, 15, 19

Valine in Hb S, 33
Vallance-Owen, J., 121
Vause, K. E., 60
Verschuer, O., 135
Victoria, Queen, 107
Viruses, 14
    cancer and, 136
    leukaemia, 69
    measles, 70
    tobacco mosaic, 18
Vitamin-D-resistant rickets, 109, 212
Vogel, F., 139

Watson, J. D., 15
Watson-Crick model of DNA, 15
Weinberg, W., 151
Whittaker, J. A., 146
Wilkins, M. H. F., 15

von Willebrand's disease, 25
Wilson's disease, 217, 218
Winiwarter, W., 56
Wiskott-Aldrich syndrome, 41, 133

X-chromatin, 73
X chromosome, 46
    deletion, 64, 79
    genes on, 50, 51, 110
    inactivation, 86, 108-109
    isochromosome formation, 79
    selection against, 165
Xeroderma pigmentosum, 132, 133
X-linked disorders, recognition of
    carriers of, 209-213
X-linked inheritance, 229
    dominant, 109
    recessive, 105-109
    in women, 108-109. *See also* Sex
    chromosomes
X-linked marker traits, 52, 211
X-linked mutations, lethal, 187, 188
Xg blood group, 109
X_m serum factor, 52

Y chromatin, 73, 74
Y chromosome, 46
    fluorescence, 74
    in Klinefelter's syndrome, 70
    in XYY syndrome, 72
Y-linked inheritance, 104, 110

Zona pellucida, 83
Zygote, 50, 83, 229